Second Journeys: The Dance of Spirit in Later Life

SECOND JOURNEYS
THE DANCE OF SPIRIT IN LATER LIFE

Bolton Anthony
EDITOR

RON PEVNY, ELLEN B. RYAN, CLAUDIA MOORE, AND RANDY MORRIS
CONTRIBUTING EDITORS

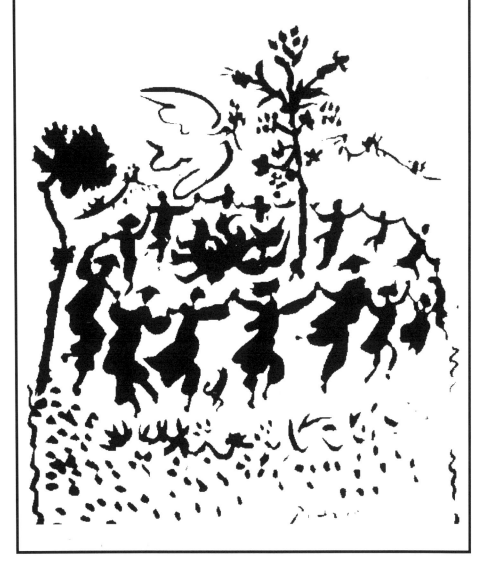

SECOND JOURNEYS

Copyright © 2013 by Second Journey Inc.

All rights reserved. No part of this publication may be reproduced or transmitted in any form or by any means, electronic or mechanical, including photocopying, recording, or any information storage or retrieval system, without prior permission. The individual articles and poems contained herein remain the intellectual property of the various authors, and permission to reproduce them, in whole or in part (except in the case of brief quotations embedded in critical articles and reviews), must be obtained from them.

Manufactured in the United States of America.

Second Journey Publications
4 Wellesley Place
Chapel Hill, NC 27517
(919) 403-0432
www.SecondJourney.org

ISBN 978-1494281090

Cover design by Michael Brady Design. Cover image is adapted from "Joie de Vivre," a lithograph by Picasso.

Interior book design by Bolton Anthony.

Table of Contents

Foreword BY JOHN G. SULLIVAN 1

Introduction BY BOLTON ANTHONY 5

Part I — Second Journeys   9

Second Journeys BY BOLTON ANTHONY 11

Fierce With Age BY CAROL ORSBORN 17

Honoring Our Elders
    Reb Zalman: Living From the Light BY ROBERT ATCHLEY 23

    The Inner Work of Eldering 26
    Selections from the Spring 2011 issue of Itineraries, with articles by Ron Pevny, Contributing Editor, Julia B. Riley, Deborah Windrum, Louden Kiracofe, and Richard Matzkin

Invitations to Practice
    Fierce with Age: The Opening Exercise BY CAROL ORSBORN 53

Part II — Aging as a Spiritual Practice   57

Excavations: A Life in Three Parts BY BOLTON ANTHONY 59

Making Room for Something New BY SARAH SUSANKA 67

Honoring Our Elders
    Connie Goldman: Mother Wisdom and the Aging Beat
    by Harry R. Moody 73

    Writing as a Spiritual Practice 76
    Selections from the Winter 2011 issue of Itineraries, with articles by Nora Zylstra-Savage, Paula Papky, Karen Bannister, and Marianne Vespry plus a new article by Contributing Editor Ellen B. Ryan

Invitations to Practice
    Writing and Aging with Spirit BY ELLEN S. JAFFE 109

Part III — Serving From Spirit   115

Remembering Christopher BY BOLTON ANTHONY 117

Peace Through Peaceful Means BY BETSY CRITES 125

Honoring Our Elders
   Dene Peterson: The Sprite of ElderSpirit by Drew Leder 135

Serving From Spirit..138
   Selections from the Summer 2011 issue of Itineraries, with articles by Claudia Moore, Contributing Editor, Edith Kusnic, Robert C. Atchley, Judith Helburn, and Pat and Steve Taylor

Invitations to Practice
   The Inner Work of Nonviolence by Betsy Crites 167

Part IV — Rites of Passage Into Elderhood — 169

The Dance of Spirit in Later Life by Bolton Anthony 171

What Are You Waiting For? by Darcy Ottey 185

Honoring Our Elders
   Fred Lanphear ~ Earth Elder by Jim Clark 191

   Rites of Passage Into Elderhood................................194
   Selections from the Fall 2011 issue of Itineraries, with articles by Harry R. Moody and John Sullivan plus a new article by Contributing Editor Randy Morris

Invitations to Practice
   Releasing the Past by Ron Pevny 225

Resources, Contributors, and Notes — 233

Reflections of a Lifelong Reader by Barbara Kammerlohr............235

About the Contributors 241

Notes..247

About Second Journey...260

Table of Contents

Listing of Poems

"The Streaker" by Bolton Anthony..................................65

"Getting There" by Lorna Louise Bell.............................162

"Cage-Free Aging" by Eugene C. Bianchi............................16

"Endings and Intimations" by Eugene C. Bianchi...................234

"Love" by John Clarke...32

"It will come to me" by Dorthi Dunsmore...........................75

"I don't do old" by Sterling Haynes..............................124

"Missing" by Phyllis Hotch.......................................100

"On Contentment" by Nina Mermey Klippel..........................246

"Construction of Time" by Grady Bennett Myers, Jr................184

"The Day Dad Died" by Ellen B. Ryan...............................52

"Now I Notice Sea Shells" by Ellen B. Ryan........................52

"The Road Now" by Ellen B. Ryan...................................79

"Iowa" by Robert Sward..86

"Sugaring" by Helen Vanier..43

"I am that old lady now" by Desiré Lyners Volkwijn................44

Listing of Book Recommendations from Selected Authors

Cecile R. Andrews, author of *Slow is Beautiful: New Visions of Community, Leisure and Joie de Vivre* 123

Angeles Arrien, author of *The Second Half of Life: Opening the Eight Gates of Wisdom*...21

Robert C. Atchley, author of *Spiritualty and Aging*..............25

Claudia Horwitz, author of *The Spiritual Activist: Practices to Transform Your Life, Your Work*.................................152

Trebbe Johnson, author of *The World Is a Waiting Lover: Desire and the Quest for the Beloved* 189

Drew Leder, author of *Spiritual Passages: Embracing Life's Sacred Journey* 133

Bill Plotkin, author of *Soulcraft: Crossing into the Mysteries of Nature and Psyche* 224

John C. Robinson, author of *The Three Secrets of Aging* 204

Ellen B. Ryan, author of the Writing Down Our Years series.........82

John Sullivan, author of *The Spiral of the Seasons: Welcoming the Gifts of Later Life*...214

Sarah Susanka, author of *The Not So Big Life: Making Room for What Really Matters* 66

Deborah Windrum, author of *Harvest the Bounty of Your Career* 38

FOREWORD
by John G. Sullivan

I have been friends with Bolton Anthony for close to 40 years. Through this new book, *Second Journeys: The Dance of Spirit in Later Life*, I meet him again and newly. Naturally, many themes persist. I think of Bolton's love of literature and poetry and film. Yet there is more. Bolton says of our mutual friend, Dene Peterson: "Her gift has been to bring so many together." In this book, Bolton does the same thing — assembling friends and encouraging them to share from their abundance.

Creation-theologian Matthew Fox begins his workshops with a circle dance. In the circle, the participants meet one another, hand to hand, face to face, in a living representation of inter-communion. Bolton, in this book, initiates the dance, or, perhaps better, reveals the dance of the Spirit in which we already move. I have enjoyed dinner parties at Bolton and Lisa's house. Often he brings folks together, saying, "I think you will like one another." And so it is here. And Bolton is present too, somewhat like the stage manager in the Thornton Wilder play *Our Town*, moving among the contributors and, from time to time, adding comments in his own voice. In Bolton's own essays, he speaks of dreams and turning points. He remembers elders who have mattered to him and trusts they will also matter to us. I think of the familiar quote: "There are no strangers, only friends we have yet to meet." Such is the mantra of one who delights, as Bolton does, in building bridges.

In these pages the reader will hear many voices and catch the resonances of many lives. Perhaps the deeper teaching is that we are not separate selves after all. When I come into the room, my parents and ancestors, my children and their children, enter with me. As do all whose gifts and wounds I bear. So the deeper teaching is that, far from being what Alan Watt stigmatized as "skin-encapsulated egos," we are, in fact, communal through and through. The many voices without remind us of the many voices within. The many voices assembled here remind us that each of us sees only partially. That we need one another. That we rise and fall together. So the watchword is to receive, to listen, heart to heart. And to return, again and again, to what my mentor, Frederick Franck called "that which matters."

In these essays, I find a fierceness. The contributors are reflecting on human lifetimes, facing the grief and anger that marks our days, facing the hurt caused by us and the hurt done to us, facing the long road to forgiveness of self and others — a long road that includes, as Reb Zalman would say, our "harsh teachers." In these essays the contributors face the wild cards that arrive in a moment — the loss of a child, the dementia of a parent — and the sudden glories as well. The contributors are fierce in facing what comes to us and to those we love — without denial, without disdain, without sentimentality. In this spirit, I am reminded that where we can relieve suffering, we seek to do so, where we can do nothing to alleviate pain, we seek to bear it together. So I find much wisdom here — how to face our lives with grace and graciousness, how to begin again and again and again.

In our time, I believe that all elders are called to be earth elders. And so the circle of life is expanded to include all the minerals and plants and animals, large and small. And we humans are included too. So I find that a spirit of oneness, of unity, shines through these essays. I see it now as a point small enough to be as close to us as we are to ourselves. I see the point now become a circle as vast as the universe and beyond. As St. Francis knew, all are our brothers and sisters — earth and water, air and fire, and even Sister Death. And we are invited to acknowledge again as did our ancestors, the native peoples, all that creates and sustains the good earth on which we stand.

Finally, I want to stay in character and end with a story:

> The tale begins in a churchyard. The narrator is talking to a gravedigger. "You know," he says, "in olden times people prayed like this" — and he spread his arms wide, involuntarily feeling his breast expand at the gesture. "In those days God would cast himself into all these human abysses, full of despair and darkness, and only reluctantly did he return into his heavens, which unnoticed, he drew

down ever closer over the earth. But a new faith began. As it could not make humans understand wherein its new God differed from their old one (for as soon as they began to praise him, they promptly recognized the one old God here too), the promulgator of the new commandment changed the manner of praying. He taught the folding of hands and declared: See, *thus* does our God wish to be implored…

Now when God next looked down upon the earth, he was frightened. Besides the many folded hands, many Gothic cathedrals had been built, and so the hands and the roofs, alike steep and sharp, stretched pointing towards him like the weapons of an enemy… God turned back into his heavens, and when he saw that the steeples and the new prayers were growing in pursuit of him, he departed out of his domain at the other side and thus eluded the chase. He was himself astonished to find, out beyond his radiant home, a beginning darkness that received him silently, and with a curious feeling he went on and on in this dusk that reminded him of the hearts of [humans].

Then for the first time it occurred to him that the heads of humans are lucid, but their hearts are full of a similar darkness; and a longing came over him to dwell in the hearts of humans and no longer to move through the clear, cold wakefulness of their thinking. Well, God has continued on his way. Ever denser grows the darkness around him, and the night through which he presses on has something of the fragrant warmth of fecund clods of earth. And in a little while the roots will reach out towards him with the old beautiful gesture of wide prayer. There is nothing wiser than the circle.[1]

Again, again we come and go,
changed, changing. Hands
join, unjoin in love and fear,
grief and joy. The circles turn,
each giving into each, into all.
Only music keeps us here,
each by all the others held.

>	from "Closing the Circle"
>	 by Wendell Berry

INTRODUCTION
by Bolton Anthony

*W*hat is the music *that "keeps us here"* in this dance of later life? What else but the *stirrings of spirit*? Spirit which draws us inward, then returns us to the world and to the circle of our fellow dancers. Spirit which in *the call to the inner work of eldering* nudges us to forsake our masks, let go of the personas we have constructed to succeed in the *business of living*, and "come home to … who we really are."[1] Spirit which in *the call to service* returns us to the "family of the earth," to those who ache for our gifts and can only survive if we join the circle and bring who we are.[2] And, paradoxically, it is only within this circle of fellow dancers — where we are "each by all the others held" — that we "discover who we are face to face and side by side with others in work, love and learning."[3]

And so the *second journey* that opens before us in later life — the invitation that comes — is a call to *mindfulness, service, and community*.

The 38 essays in this anthology explore this "dance of spirit in later life." The book's four sections — Second Journeys, Aging as a Spiritual Practice, Serving from Spirit, and Rites of Passage Into Elderhood — mirror the thematic organization of the four issues of *Itineraries* published during our yearlong exploration of The Spirituality of Later Life. Throughout the book, new essays companion selections from the original 2011 series. Each of the four sections contains a tribute to an elder whose life has been emblematic, and each concludes with an "Invitation to Practice."

Interspersed throughout the book, a number of authors who have been our *virtual partners* in this effort to birth a new vision of aging for our time offer brief reflections on the books which have sustained and nourished them in their own efforts. The many poems, scattered through the book, invite you to linger and reflect. Finally, Barbara Kammerlohr, who has long served as book reviewer for Second Journey, offers her recommendations for further reading and exploration.

I FOUNDED SECOND JOURNEY some 14 years ago, when I was 55. It grew out of a vague idea that at that point was itself over a decade old, a concept I called Centers for Imagining the Future. My work with the 1898 centennial commemoration in Wilmington, North Carolina, was ending. What should I do next? If I didn't follow now where this idea led, would the future hold another chance?

As a way of pondering the decision, I took a road trip, meeting with a number of people — some old friends, some new. The trip took me to Mike Callaghan's home, a sculptor, potter, and dear, now-departed friend of many years. I had always traced the birth of the idea back to the physical space Mike had created in his home below Hanging Rock, where one wall of a womb-like living room is a magnificent 20-foot-high clunk of that ancient mountain.

Toward the end of our conversation, Mike said, —You should just do it.
—Do what?
—Do the Center. Just start it. Start one concrete place.

I shared this advice farther down the road with another friend, Morgan Adams, and she concurred. She was, however, talking about the "Virtual Community of Inquiry" — starting that dialogue around which one or more concrete places would coalesce. But she also thought I should simply "do it."

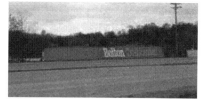

I was thinking about the decision the next day. My son Thomas and I were on our way to Mammoth Cave, where we planned to spend the afternoon, before going on to Cincinnati to see my daughter Andrea in a play. I was driving through southern rural Kentucky in the early morning. On the outskirts of a small town named Somerset, I came around a curve in the road and saw …

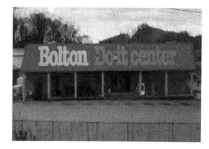

So, I have "done it." Or, to speak with more accuracy, WE have done it.

Introduction

THERE ARE MANY, MANY PEOPLE to thank. The 45 contributors of the essays and poems which appear in this book are joined by more than 150 others who have honored us by allowing their work to be published in *Itineraries* during this past decade. Ron Pevny, Ellen Ryan, and Randy Morris, who all shepherded separate issues of the 2011 series to publication, have each contributed new pieces to the book. Our fourth Contributing Editor, Claudia Moore, succumbed recently to a serious illness and is missed. These four, also, are representatives of another dozen or more Guest Editors who over the years played similar roles with specific issues of *Itineraries*. It's fitting to acknowledge and honor the recent work of Penelope Bourk, Janice Blanchard, and Gaya Erlandson. To all these many generous and talented people, I offer my deep and heartfelt thanks.

For the past nine years, I have been companioned in these endeavors by my wife, Lisa, who, in addition to the usual encouragement and support for which wives are usually thanked, played the role of professional copyeditor, uncompromisingly insisting on a standard of near perfection. I thank her for all her many hours of uncompensated work and for her devoted love.

*Think of these [extra years of life] as a resource
— a cultural and spiritual resource reclaimed
from death in the same way the Dutch reclaim fertile
land from the waste of the sea. During any one of
those years, somebody who no longer has to worry
about raising a family, pleasing a boss,*

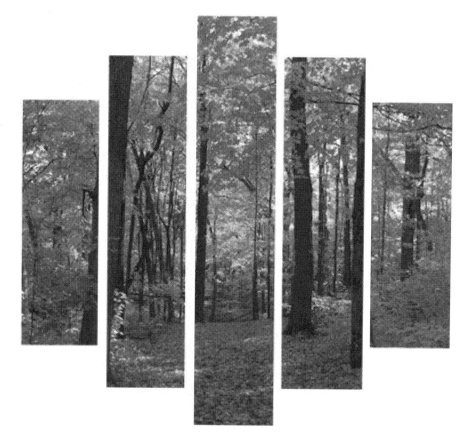

*or earning more money will have the chance to join
with others in building a compassionate society where
people can think deep thoughts, create beauty, study
nature, teach the young, worship what they hold
sacred, and care for one another.*
— THEODORE ROSZAK

PART I

SECOND JOURNEYS

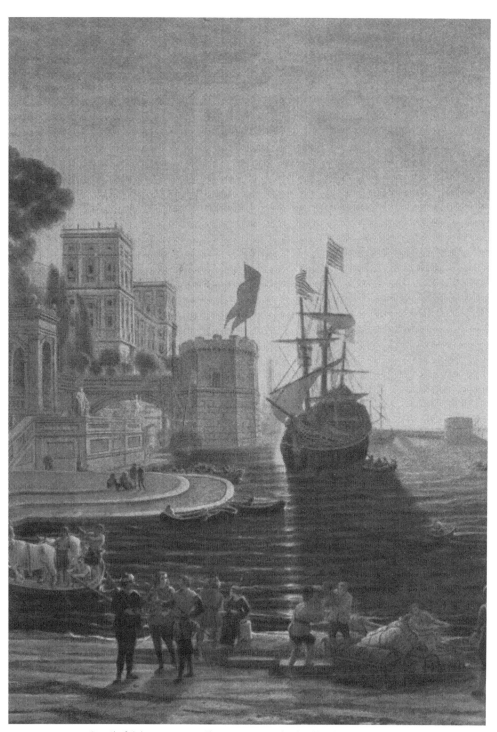
Detail of *Odysseus returns Chryseis to Her Father* by Claude Lorrain (circa 1644)

The poet Tennyson imagines Ulysses, the hero of that great poem of homecoming, *The Odyssey*, chafing in his old age for another great adventure:

> How dull it is to pause, to make an end,
> To rust unburnished, not to shine in use!
> As though to breathe were life.[1]

He will leave the "scepter and the isle" — the task of administering the kingdom — to his son Telemachus. Though governance has traditionally been the province of old men (hence the word "senator" from the Latin root *sen* meaning old), Ulysses lacks the disposition for it, the "slow prudence" needed "to make mild/ A rugged people, and through soft degrees / Subdue them to the useful and the good."

SECOND JOURNEYS

BY BOLTON ANTHONY

The call that Ulysses feels is to the *heroic*, to an intensity of life that is available only to those *warriors* who, with comrades, engage in some death-defying struggle of great moment. He is old; he and his fellow mariners "are not now that strength which in old days / Moved earth and heaven." And yet…

> Old age hath yet his honor and his toil.
> … but something ere the end,
> Some work of noble note, may yet be done,
> Not unbecoming men that strove with Gods.

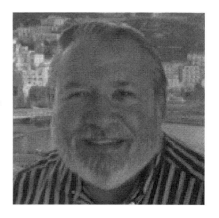

And so, Tennyson — in this *prelude* to an *unrecounted* second journey — imagines Ulysses and his crew setting out, poised "to sail beyond the sunset, and the baths / Of all the western stars" — firm in conviction that it is "not too late to seek a newer world."

The poetry is stirring. Never mind that this call to *shine in use* is made to comrades in arms who have "drunk delight of battle with [their] peers." Robert Kennedy, who took no delight in war and struggled valiantly to end one, chose the title for his book, *To Seek a Newer World*, from among Tennyson's lines as he sought to rouse a generation to action. Might not this same generation — now themselves "made weak by time and fate" — find here renewed inspiration and rekindled idealism for their own second journeys? But what *kind* of second journey?

The suggestion that a further adventure awaits the aging Ulysses occurs midway through *The Odyssey*, when he encounters the blind seer Tiresias at the border of Hades. After prophesying — *accurately* — the many trials and years of wandering that will precede Ulysses' reunion with Penelope, Tiresias tells him of this later journey:

> …not a sea journey, although he must carry with him a well-cut oar. Turning inland he must travel on until he reaches a country where the people have never seen the sea… [H]e will recognize the right place when he meets a stranger, who, seeing the oar, will ask him about the "winnowing fan" he is carrying on his shoulder.[2]

The Odyssey as it comes down to us from Homer concludes without this promised epilogue. We must wait two millennia for another great poet, Dante, "to imagine in unforgettable lines" the subsequent voyage that is the inspiration for Tennyson's poem:

> [his] final sailing beyond the pillars of the western world… towards the southern pole… until [he sees] on the horizon a great mountain rising out of the seas towards heaven. With cries of eagerness [he urges his] crew towards it, but there comes a huge wave rolling from the mountain, becoming a whirlpool as it sucks [his] ship, [him]self and all [his] companions down into the depths to join the shades below.[3]

For what Dante apparently considered reckless arrogance, Ulysses is consigned to the eighth circle of hell.

When I founded Second Journey in 1999, it was the second journey in another work of imaginative literature — *Narcissus and Goldmund* by the twentieth-century German novelist Hermann Hesse — that suggested the name I gave the organization.

Near the end of that book, Hesse imagines his aging protagonist, Goldmund — exhausted after the completion of his masterwork — embarking on an adventure meant to reprise his coming-of-age journey. The journey is an unqualified disaster. Goldmund, who is thrown from his horse and injured within a day's ride of the monastery he has left, is prevented only by pride from dragging himself back. He soldiers on only to discover that the charms of his youth have deserted him, and the young women he would woo find his advances abhorrent. Months later, broken in health, he returns to the monastery — to die.[4]

The temptation to which Goldmund, like Ulysses, yields is to try *to repeat himself*: to live the second half of life as he had the first — to rely on that same repertoire of skills that had served him well, not recognizing that some tectonic shift had occurred in his life. We spend the first half of our lives creating an *ego* that allows us to "succeed" in the world — building on the *strengths* that allow us to make a life, raise a family, have a career, or, at minimum, just survive for 50 years. Then we cross some sort of boundary and enter an undiscovered country where all the accustomed wiles and ways of our ego seem ineffectual. Girded for another sea adventure, we find ourselves sloughing through a pathless jungle with no view of the night sky and the canopy of stars we used to steer by.

Carl Jung thought in later life we were forced to deal with the world not from our strengths, but from our *weaknesses*, from out of what he called our *shadow*. Does the ego, this fine and efficient distillation of our life experience, have to *die*? And if so, to make way for what?

A dream I had when I turned 50 has helped me think about these matters. In the dream, I was a screenwriter who'd been asked by a producer (in whose debt I was) to try to rescue a project he feared had become hopelessly mired. I was to work with the director, whose earlier work I knew and admired; but he was an old man now, and many years had elapsed since his last film. We spent the day together walking about the set; and I found, as I listened to the director talk about the film, I was listening less to *what* he said than to *who* he was.

At the end of the day we somehow arrived at the vestibule of his home. He had been speaking when I interrupted him:

> "I have decided what I will do," I told him. "I'll rewrite those scenes where I think there are problems and make my best case for the changes. If — after you've looked thoughtfully at my suggestions

— you still think things should be handled differently, then I'll write it however you wish." *Why?* I thought, but did not say. Because I trust you. Because I trust that you know where this needs to go.

It is not that our carefully honed skills of a lifetime, our many strengths, are useless; it is rather that they must be put *in service to something larger than the ego* (which is always the "I" in our dreams). The Tiresias in each of us, that sage towards whom we are journeying, knows *exactly* what it wants.

My words to the director, my *decision* to help to him, were perhaps triggered by the words of reassurance he'd just spoken. The "vestibule" in which we stood was a constricted courtyard, enclosed by high cement block walls. Against one of its walls, a single rose bush was espaliered. My guide had detected the dread which the austere and sterile courtyard — this threshold between midlife and elderhood — had created in me. He'd sought to allay my fears, inviting me into his lovely home where his beautiful wife waited to welcome me — inviting me into this next stage of life.

In her insightful essay on *The Odyssey* from which I quoted above, Helen Luke weaves the sparse details found in Homer — the journey overland to a remote interior village whose inhabitants "have never seen the sea," the "well-cut oar" that will be mistaken for a "winnowing fan" — into an illuminating parable that describes the journey into elderhood.

A restless longing for adventure and glory — the desire to discover new lands and sail unknown seas — grows again in the aging Ulysses:

> Slowly and unconsciously the arrogance that had caused his long sufferings [during his first journey home from Troy] returned — working, as it always does, through the best of his human qualities — through his longing to know and to see all the wonders of creation and to understand things as yet hidden from most men.[5]

These burgeoning plans to reprise his earlier journey are, however, suddenly cut short when the seer Tiresias comes to him again in a dream, reminding him of the alternate, inland journey which Ulysses realizes he has somehow "completely blotted out from his conscious mind."

The dream prompts a kind of *life review*. He recognizes the "foolish arrogance" that characterized his dealing with the Cyclops. He sees how "puffed up with his own cleverness" he had been and how his crew had paid dearly with their lives for his ego inflation. He feels shame for his actions, and a deep compassion grows in him for those he had wronged so grievously.[6]

The next day, he sets out alone — a small donkey carrying his provisions and the oar — on a journey that becomes for Luke a beautiful metaphor for the journey into elderhood. Ulysses does not understand — "not yet," she adds — and yet he *obeys*. "One thing was clear — this journey would bring no glory." This was a journey into the *interior*, which held little interest to seafaring men of action. This was a journey into the depths, where "there were no maps to follow once he came to the last known village... [and] he must simply walk on into the unknown."

A winnowing fan is the tool used by farmers to separate the wheat from the chaff:

> ...a process that mirrors in the psychic realm the acquisition of wisdom and mature judgment, the ability to discern between that which really matters and that which doesn't. According to [Luke's] interpretation, Odysseus isn't simply being asked to retire and renounce his power and prowess, he is being asked to exchange it for that which he has learned along the way, the wisdom to weigh alternatives and discard the less desirable ones. In short, this last journey really is an *elderquest* because its successful completion requires the mastery of a whole new set of skills, those that are necessary to navigate not midlife but old age — trust, wisdom, and the willingness to let go.[7]

So, extending to you the gesture of welcome the director in my film made, I invite you to embark upon your own second journey. It is a journey into the interior, into the unfamiliar — a journey that will require the kind of inner work described in the essays which follow. It is also — paradoxically — a journey which will return you to service in the world: "Go far enough on the inner journey, [the great wisdom traditions] all tell us — go past ego toward true self — and you end up not lost in narcissism but returning to the world, bearing more gracefully the responsibilities that come with being human."[8]

Trust that what awaits you is a second homecoming in the house of wisdom "where the people who love you are waiting."[9]

Cage-Free Aging

Chickens scratch and cluck
happy to rub beaks and wink
freed by Amish farmers in praise of God.
I'd like to think my eighty-one goes freer,
smiling more at college chicks
who brighten back unthreatened by grandfather's gray.
Old cages played their part with memories sweet
of books, student faces, even former wives
and priests and deans setting borders,
dispensing rules and nostrums from every side.
I struggled to set life in a long row of respectable confinements
for maximum product and praise,
longing to sit secure at the right hand
of the Grand Cager in that blessed caging
watching his deputies pace the perimeters
for our everlasting good.
Most of us cage-dwellers mean well
as we embrace familiar limits
and hesitate before open doors
to sniff the air blown from places unknown,
afraid to jump down to grass wet with surprise.
Now with a view from age,
I delight in modest leaps
toward freedom and joy.

— Eugene C. Bianchi[†]

[†] From *Ear to the Ground: Poems from the Long View* by Eugene C. Bianchi (Parson's Porch Publishers, 2013).

I've got an invitation for you that you won't be able to refuse. It's a multiyear, in-depth course that is designed to strip away your ego, confront you with ultimate questions about meaning and purpose, and give you the opportunity to come to terms with mortality while learning to appreciate the present moment.

It's called aging.

If you are fortunate to live long enough, you won't have a choice about whether or not you will be confronted with losses, challenges, and diminishments that accompany growing older. You *will* have the opportunity to choose whether you will become a victim of age or, alternately, transform aging into a spiritual path that at last offers the promise of fulfilling your true human potential.

FIERCE WITH AGE

BY CAROL ORSBORN

When I refer to aging as a spiritual path, let me be clear. I'm not just talking about peace and serenity here. On the contrary, conscious elderhood demands a level of commitment that often seems to require more of us than we think we have to give. For starters, we need to fight the ageist images of growing older that we, ourselves, have internalized. We need to confront, grapple with, and ultimately transcend the dread and even revulsion that has sadly become the hallmark of the mainstream attitude about aging. Coupled with this, we must simultaneously resist the urge to romanticize or whitewash aging, defying an antiaging society's denial of both the realities and promise that is the truth about growing old.

Central to this is questioning the myth of "serenity" as the chief characteristic and goal of what is known in the gerontology field as "successful aging." To place serenity in its contemporary context, we need only trace its modern-day origins to the years following World War II. During the war, the young men went to battlefields around the world, leaving women and the elderly behind to keep the home front functioning. Older people and women worked the

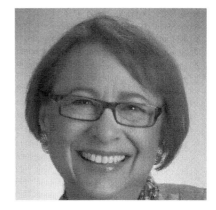

fields, ran the factories, and stepped up into leadership roles in every industry. At war's end, it became their patriotic duty to step aside to make room for the returning warriors. In its place, Madison Avenue offered older folks the promise of romanticized suburbs, gated communities, and retirements of leisure — on the golf course or in a rocking chair. The "geezers" who resisted marginalization were portrayed as "eccentric" or "disloyal." Serenity, in other words, was a way of marginalizing and dismissing older people. Serene people, after all, "make no trouble" and slip graciously out of sight and mind.

Of course, there is a place for serenity in our lives. But the mystics of many traditions have a much broader understanding of what it means to walk that spiritual path. While I have been a lifelong student of mystical and spiritual literature from a broad range of traditions, it wasn't until I was personally confronted with my own aging and mortality that I transcended both the dread of growing older as well as romanticized fantasies of the future and replaced them with a more prophetic relationship to the divine. There are still times, of course, when I am quiet and peaceful. But I have learned that with six decades behind me, I am rabble-rousing more than ever. I am not above standing on the mountain top and shaking my fist at God, nor do I think there's something wrong with me when I have sunk into the dark night of the soul. I have come to realize that as long as we keep growing, there will be anxious moments, regrets, and self-doubt. But there will be transiting, transforming, and overcoming, too. As a result, I have put being at peace farther down on the list of aspirations as I age. At the top is to be fully alive, no matter the consequences. This is the essence of what I refer to when I describe my current orientation towards life as having become "fierce with age."

This knowledge was hard won for me. In my recent memoir, *Fierce with Age: Chasing God and Squirrels in Brooklyn,*[1] I recorded the ups and downs of a tumultuous year spent facing, busting, and ultimately triumphing over the stereotypes of aging. Having landed a yearlong project in New York too good to refuse, my husband Dan had enticed me away from my beloved cottage in a Los Angeles canyon to move to a high-rise apartment in Brooklyn. As the year unfolded, I nurtured a love-starved friend through a doomed affair with a younger man, dealt with my own physical and social changes, and sought to regain my passion for life at the side of my squirrel-crazed dog, Lucky. One of the most disconcerting challenges I faced was that in the process of transiting out of my comfort zone and into the wild space beyond midlife, I'd somehow forgotten who I was and how to restore my faith in life.

One moment, I'd been a smart, high-achieving spiritual woman at the peak of her game. The next moment, it was as if I had forgotten everything I'd learned over the course of my life. Shockingly out of control, I could not get things to go back the way they were, complete a grieving process, or martial my internal and external resources to greet a life-threatening diagnosis. Apparently, I had entered a new, prolonged life stage: one that our entire society — in an effort to trivialize the stage — either denies, reviles, or sentimentalizes. In short, I had become old.

I learned a lot about myself, aging, and life over the course of the year. And as our year in New York was coming to an end, once again surrounded by packing boxes, I found myself with my faith renewed. Because of everything I endured, I began this new phase of my life journey no longer ashamed or depleted about aging — curious and excited instead. While the contours of this wild terrain beyond midlife have not yet fully revealed themselves to me, I am clear that rather than experiencing myself at an ending, I have most definitively embarked upon something profoundly and unexpectedly new.

Happily, I am not alone. We have role models who hail from a broad range of religious and spiritual communities who are pointing the way. Here's a wonderful quote from Henri Nouwen: "Aging is the gradual fulfillment of the life cycle in which receiving matures in giving and living makes dying worthwhile. Aging does not need to be hidden or denied, but can be understood, affirmed, and experienced as a process of growth by which the mystery of life is slowly revealed to us…The elderly are our prophets, they remind us that what we see so clearly in them is a process in which we all share."[2]

John C. Robinson, in his illuminating *The Three Secrets of Aging: A Radical Guide*, asks, "What if people began to experience age-related changes in consciousness as essentially mystical in nature?"[3] Harry R. Moody writes, "In the most profound mystical tradition, the way of transcendence entails at its highest point the 'loss of the self.'"[4] You will find prophetic assertions equating aging with fulfillment in writings of Rabbi Zalman Schachter-Shalomi, Sister Joan Chittister, Buddhist priest Lewis Richmond, and many more.

I leaned heavily on these and many other pioneers of the conscious aging movement while I was in the heat of my own transition to the wild side of midlife. And in the months following, I felt called to draw upon all my skills as a scholar (with a doctorate in religion and masters of theological studies), teacher, spiritual counselor, and retreat leader to help others utilize their own psychological and spiritual resources to more fully re-vision what this age and stage of our lives can mean for us.

Central to the spiritual practice of aging is a common theme: letting go of the illusion of control. Of course, most of us prefer the notion that we are calling the shots in our lives, applying ourselves to making things turn out the way we want, and feeling that we have mastery over our circumstances. But, the daunting part about aging is this: Some and eventually all of our old tricks no longer work. We realize how much of our sense of mastery over our fates has always been limited, at best.

As it turns out, when viewed through the lens of psychological and spiritual maturity, this is a good thing, Virtually every spiritual and religious philosophy centers on the shattering of illusions — be it the Hebrews tearing down false idols or the Buddhists seeing through the maya of surface manifestation. When we strip away the impositions, the fantasies, and the denial, we begin to view aging as holding the potential for activation of new, unprecedented levels of self-affirmation, meaning, and spiritual growth.

As I said earlier, this psychologically and spiritually healthy vision of aging does not feel like serenity. *The truth is, as long as we keep growing through life, there will be anxious moments, regrets, and self-doubt. But there will be transiting, transforming, and overcoming, too.*

In place of the stereotypes of aging, this prophetic vision of aging beckons us to take into account both the light and the shadow side of growing old, neither romanticizing nor reviling the years beyond midlife. This is no small order. In fact, waking up to ultimate concerns while maintaining both a hopeful and realistic vision of the aging process requires a level of spiritual maturity that is a challenge to the best of us. But it is also the stripping away of illusion and a thinning of the veil between our ordinary lives and the divine. This is the essence of the mystical path: the promise of aging as the fulfillment of our true human potential. In fact, rather than dreading age, we have the opportunity to become fierce with age.

As a cultural anthropologist, I have observed that a point of unity that humankind shares is the experience of transcendence. The heart of my own spiritual journey has been shaped by the ancient roots of mysticism and perennial wisdoms found in all spiritual traditions. Additionally, I have been deeply influenced by the splendor and restorative power of Nature.

The books that I continue to return to are: Evelyn Underhill's classic, *Mysticism*, and Wayne Teasdale's *The Mystic Heart*. Besides Thoreau's *Walden* and *The Wisdom of the Wilderness* by Gerald May, I consistently read poet Mary Oliver whose writing is filled with gratitude about daily encounters with nature. *Essential Spirituality* by Roger Walsh and *Shadows of the Sacred* by Frances Vaughan describe what is both essential and challenging within the spiritual journey. Favorite sources of spiritual solace and inspiration are John O'Donohue's *Eternal Echoes* and Huston Smith's *The World's Religions*.

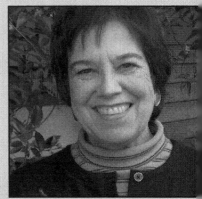

Angeles Arrien

Angeles Arrien is a cultural anthropologist, award-winning author, educator, and consultant to many organizations and businesses. She lectures and conducts workshops worldwide, bridging cultural anthropology, psychology, and comparative religions. Her work currently is used in medical, academic, and corporate environments. Angeles is the President of the Foundation for Cross-Cultural Education and Research. Her seven books have been translated into 13 languages, and she has received three honorary doctorate degrees in recognition of her work. She is the author of the contemporary classics, *The Four-Fold Way* and *The Second Half of Life*, which won the 2007 Nautilus Award for Best Book on Aging. Her latest book, *Living in Gratitude: A Journey that will Change Your Life*, was recognized as one of the Best Spiritual Books of 2011.

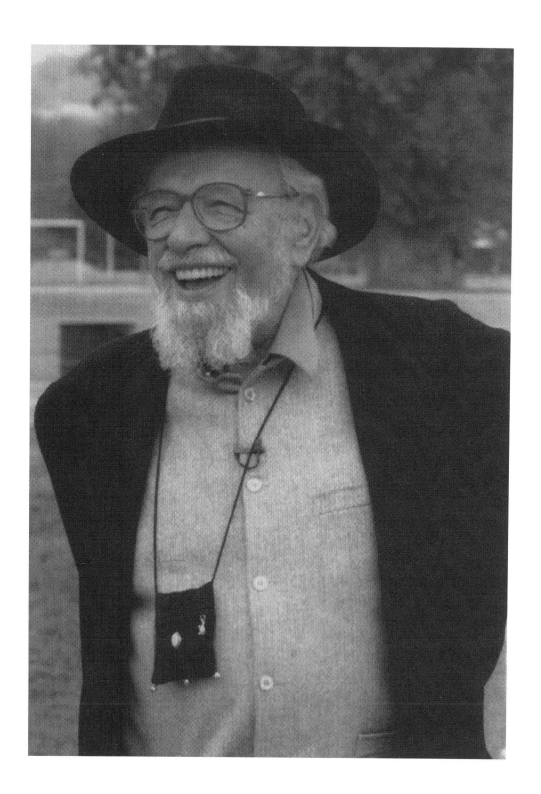

Honoring Our Elders

Reb Zalman: Living from the Light

Many of our ideas about aging with consciousness have their origins in the life and thought of Rabbi Zalman Schachter-Shalomi, called "Reb Zalman" by the many thousands whose lives have been deeply affected by his ideas and presence. Reb Zalman's writings, especially *From Age-ing to Sage-ing: A Profound New Vision of Growing Older*, and his workshops on "Spiritual Eldering" have provided a stimulating conceptual overview of how we might think about spiritual growth in later life — how we might think, in particular, about our potential for spiritual connection and our capacity to manifest wisdom, and their importance at all levels of social life. But as useful as his ideas have been, Reb Zalman's way of being and its ongoing evolution is perhaps his greatest lesson for us.

In my own spiritual journey, I have met many people who are so in touch with the sacred that a holy light radiates from them. Reb Zalman is one of these. He makes no claim to have answers to life's churning conveyor belt of perplexing questions. Instead, he contemplates the deeper questions and affords them the largest possible space in which to reveal their lessons. This contemplative space within his consciousness allows Reb Zalman to balance a keen, creative, and active mind with an extraordinarily open heart and deep knowledge of the history of human wisdom. He is continuously learning from deeply contemplated life experience.

Living proof that if we encourage people to be wise they can be, he has honed his "wisdom process" over decades of listening deeply to people who come seeking wisdom from him. "I am not wise until someone asks me to be," he has said. Wisdom is not something to have, it is something to be in a given moment. Of course, the more often people practice being wise, the more likely they are to be able to find that place within themselves from which wisdom comes. And Reb Zalman has had lots of practice.

I attend a discussion group with Reb Zalman that has been meeting weekly for more than a decade. We explore such issues as the frontiers of spiritual experience and spiritual development, and examine whether spirituality can influence the world, and if so how, in discussions that range far and wide. Reb Zalman knows how to listen with compassion, to be open to both the joy and the pain underlying whatever is said. He also knows that singing and humor are vital glue that helps groups stick together. He is a repository of wisdom stories from many spiritual traditions and a master of using them to help us see an important side of the issue under discussion. His stories remind us that spiritually grounded wisdom has been a part of human life for a very long time. They press us to think through the implications of our spiritual insights for action on many levels — family, community, nation, and planet.

Reb Zalman's own life is structured around the demands of his own religious devotion, and he is always a Rabbi. But he is a Rabbi who understands his role as one that is consciously re-created in the moment rather than dictated from an unchanging script. Although a devout Jew, he honors all religious traditions, holding that all were initially inspired by the same Light.

Reb Zalman is an exemplar of someone who lives from the Light, someone who is never far from direct contact with the Light of being. Even when he feels lost, he trusts that he will return to the Light. It is an irresistible magnet for him. His life is an uncommonly well-documented struggle to remain true to the Light, while still leading an ordinary human life. Like all of us, he has to deal with the ups and downs that come with living in an aging body, being part of a family, living in a community, and so on. For Reb Zalman, keeping in touch with the sacred Light is a source of optimism with which to resist the powers of darkness that often seem to be overtaking our world.

In honoring our elders, we not only honor who they are for us, we honor the potential for spiritual connection and wisdom within ourselves. Our elders point the way, but we each have to find our own inner path.

— Robert C. Atchley

One book? You've got to be kidding. I'm a book guy, always in search of better ways to write about that which can't really be written about. My library of "holy books" contains more than 50 much-used volumes. My first glimmer into mystical reality came from *On the Road*, by Jack Kerouac. It was existentialism — the Now — subtly wrapped in Hindu philosophy. *I Am That: Dialogues with Nisargadatta Maharaj* uses a Socratic method to unveil the ultimate reality that lives within us all. This book led me to India, to my spiritual "advanced graduate program" with Maharaj, and I can never forget his simple teaching — pay full attention to pure being and everything else will become clear. For poets, *Anam Chara* by John O'Donohoe, is a marvelous book about spiritual relationship. Finally, the book I carry with me most often is *Stillness Speaks* by Eckhart Tolle. This thin volume is full of reminders for those of us who have been on the path for awhile. I can open it to a random page and after a little reading I stop and am drawn away from my mind into just being, into peaceful waiting. Not waiting for anything, just hanging out with what is happening, no thoughts.

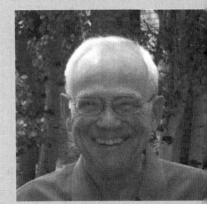

Robert Atchley

Bob Atchley is author of *Spirituality and Aging*, *Continuity and Adaptation in Aging*, *Social Forces and Aging* and 25 other books. He is also a singer-songwriter whose recorded songs include "The Journey," "Pay Close Attention," "When We Come Home," "We're Awake," "Searching for Soul," and many others. Currently he is involved with Second Journey, Sage-ing® International, and the Legacy of Wisdom Project.

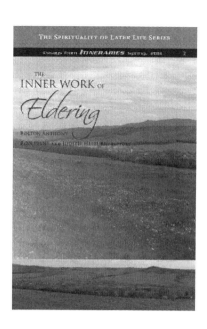

THE INNER WORK OF ELDERING

2011 Spring issue of *Itineraries:* Selections and Supplements

The Fruits of Conscious Eldering
    by Ron Pevny, Contributing Editor 27

Forgiveness... The Gift You Give Yourself
    by Julia B. Riley.. 33

Honoring the Cycles of Our Inner Seasons
    by Deborah Windrum 39

The Epiphany of Life-Altering Illnesses
    by Louden Kiracofe... 45

Artistic Creativity As Renewal in Eldering
    by Richard Matzkin... 49

The Fruits of Conscious Eldering

by **Ron Pevny**, Contributing Editor

ON ONE OF THE CONSCIOUS ELDERING retreats that I lead, a participant in her early sixties shared something that had a powerful impact on all present. In reflecting on her intentions for her retreat, she spoke of two significant older people in her life. One, who was in relatively good physical health, was difficult to be around because of her seemingly constant anger, bitterness, and negativity. She was old and miserable. People avoided her because she was a drain on their energy and joy. The other was a woman who, while not physically healthy, attracted people like a magnet. In her presence they felt joy, serenity, optimism, peace. People saw her as an elder whose radiance and wisdom lifted their spirits. Our retreat participant affirmed her intention, on this retreat and on her journey ahead, to grow into a radiant elder rather than a joyless old person; and she shared her questions and concerns about how to accomplish this.

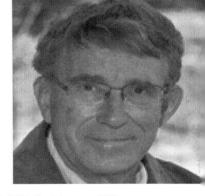

The aging process seems to bring out either the worst or the best in people — magnifying and emphasizing the flaws and shadow elements of some of us; amplifying the wisdom, radiance, and compassion in others. The question carried by those of us committed to becoming peaceful, fulfilled elders is, "How can my aging bring out the best in me?" The inner work known by rubrics such as "conscious eldering," "conscious aging," "spiritual eldering," and "Sage-ing" holds important answers to this question.

The journey from late middle-age into fulfilled elderhood is facilitated by inner work that is focused and fueled by conscious intention. This journey can lead to the pinnacle of one's emotional and spiritual development. Undertaking this journey is in fact what our lives to that point have prepared us for. And as conscious elders, our service to our communities and to the community of all beings can be profound. Carl Jung succinctly expressed this potential: "A human being would certainly not grow to be seventy or eighty years old if this longevity had no meaning for the species. The afternoon of human life must also have a significance of its own…"[1]
The word *conscious* is key to understanding the wide range of ways that the inner work of eldering may be done. It is also key to the distinction

between being "old" and being an "elder." Conscious means aware. Aware of who we really are, of our authentic emotions, talents, aspirations, strengths, and weaknesses. Aware of a growth process unfolding in our lives through all of our experiences, positive and painful. Aware of that within us which is conditioned by the myriad of disempowering messages that surround us, as well as that which is authentic, natural, and life supporting. Aware of those shadow elements in us — our dark sides — which can block our radiance and sabotage our potential.

Life Review

If the essence of conscious eldering is increasing awareness, then its core practice is Life Review. "Wisdom does not come from having experiences," as my colleagues in Sage-ing® International frequently remind me. "Wisdom comes from reflecting on one's life experiences." There are many ways of doing Life Review. Some entail *structured exercises* to focus on challenges, learning, and growth during the stages of one's life; and they use pen, computer, or art materials as tools. *Oral history work* with a knowledgeable friend or guide can be a powerful catalyst for remembering life experiences and discovering their significance. The grandmother of a colleague of mine creatively memorialized key events in the life of her family by creating a "family quilt" over a period of many years. Whichever method most resonates with us, what is critical is doing it. The awareness we gain is what makes virtually all the other inner work possible and effective. The elder wisdom we arrive at is a precious gift to the descendants who will remember us.

Healing the Past

Much of the inner work of eldering focuses on healing and letting go of old baggage. Actualizing our unique potential as elders requires that our energy be free and clear, that our psyches be capable of embracing the possibilities and opportunities of each present moment rather than stuck in the experiences of the past. We can't shine as radiant elders if our energy is continually sapped by old wounds, grudges, angers, hurts, and feelings of victimhood. We can't move lightly and serenely through our days when we have not forgiven others or ourselves for the slights and hurts we have experienced and perpetrated through unconscious behavior. We cannot display our wholeness when unprocessed grief keeps open wounds that sap our energy.

When we review our lives, we become aware of the immense power of story. We become aware of the myths we have constructed for our lives as the result of our experiences — the stories we tell ourselves (and oftentimes others) about our lives that shape who we become as the years pass. We see how disempowering these stories can be when they contain strong motifs of victimhood, inadequacy, unworthiness, and regret. It is liberating to know that the stories can be changed and that doing so is perhaps the most powerful inner work we can do as we age. This process is often called "recontextualizing" or "reframing."

Recontextualizing

The essence of recontextualizing is viewing painful or difficult life experiences with the intention of finding what in those experiences has contributed — or has the potential now to contribute, as we reappropriate it with conscious awareness — to our growth and learning. Taking a longer view of our lives, the job we lost may have pushed us into a difficult search that led to a fuller expression of our gifts. The wounding inflicted on us by another may have taught us compassion or empathy for the suffering of others. The hurt we inflicted on another may have been a teacher for us about our shadow side — a critical awareness if we are to grow as human beings. A career decision we made that we regret may have been a crucial step toward our becoming who we are today, even if the mechanics of this are not obvious.

Recontextualizing experiences that do not hold a strong emotional charge can be relatively easy. But if this practice is to truly impact our lives at the level of deep feeling and allow us to reshape the stories we live by, then we must grapple with emotionally charged experiences, allow ourselves to deeply feel suppressed emotion, and do the inner work of forgiving or grieving. At its core, recontextualizing is profoundly spiritual work. It requires a deep trust that the divine intelligence present in us has a purpose for our lives and is working through our experiences to achieve that purpose. We may not understand its workings, and they may not be what we would choose. But this wise inner guidance possesses the eagle's eye view of our lives that eludes the narrower view of our ego selves.

Deepening Spiritual Connection

Our ability to trust in a divine intelligence with a purpose for our lives depends greatly upon the strength of our connection to a Higher Power — to Spirit, Soul, God, the Great Mystery. The inner work of eldering requires us to find spiritual practices that nurture that connection. The goal of all true spiritual practice is, of course, to help us experience ourselves and our lives in a wider context, framed in a truer story than the stories our ego selves tend to create about our lives. When we trust — with a trust grounded in the deep inner knowing that flows from spiritual connection — that our lives have prepared us to become wise elders, our unfolding stories become gifts to our communities.

Our deepening spiritual connection is intrinsically related to the shift from a life grounded in "doing" to one grounded in "being" — a shift that is a key dynamic in conscious eldering. When we make this shift we move from living and acting with the primary goal of meeting the needs of our ego selves, to living and acting so that Spirit (or however we may name it) shines through us as fully as possible.

Accepting Mortality

The world's great spiritual traditions consistently teach us that accepting our mortality is perhaps our biggest ally in helping us to truly embrace life and the wonder of each moment. Yet we live amid pervasive denial of mortality. Illness and physical loss — realities for most of us as we age — have great power to transform denial into an acceptance that gives zest to each of our limited number of days.

Creating Legacy

We all leave a legacy — positive, negative, or mixed — to the generations that follow us. Aging consciously requires that we become aware of the legacy we have created up to this point in our lives and intentional about the legacy we want to create in our elderhood. Life review and the work of bringing healing to the past help us acknowledge and build on the positives of this evolving legacy and free up the energy needed to identify and move forward in building the legacy that is our gift to the future. Here again, a growing spiritual connection that allows us to see clearly our unique calling and gifts as an elder is key. This *experience* of a calling, or vocation, helps us become aware of the legacy we truly want to leave and of the path that will help us realize this goal. It opens our heart, strengthens our intention, focuses our action, and taps our spiritual depths so that we bring our *whole* selves to the creation of legacy.

Letting Go

We cannot move fully from who we have been into the elder we can become without letting go of that which will not support us on this journey. We all have culturally instilled attitudes and beliefs about life and aging that are disempowering. Our inner work is to become *conscious* (aware) of these and then to let them go. We all have attachments to people, places, things, activities, ideologies, attitudes, old stories, and self-identifications that may (or may not) have served us in the past but which will definitely not serve us in the future. Here again, our work is awareness and surrender. Life review is a valuable tool in becoming aware of what must be surrendered.

Rituals of letting go, whether conducted alone or with the support and witness of a group, can be powerful tools for transforming that awareness into willingness to let go of who we have been. Intentional rites of passage in elderhood — initiatory rituals — can allow us to let go of outworn identifications. True, effective surrender requires a deep trust that by letting go of the familiar and what has come to feel "safe," albeit constricting, we are supported by the wisdom and life force which is calling us into a new identity and positive new beginnings.

While the inner work of eldering is "work" — at times quite difficult work — it is also dynamic and enlivening. It can be the most important work we ever do. It may well be accompanied by tears of both sadness and joy, as bound-up energies are freed to reflect a growing consciousness of who we are and what is possible. Its fruits can be the radiance, passion, and service so needed by a world in need of conscious elders. We wish you well on your journey.

Love

Let go, let go.
Love will hold on still.

We slowly see
the rock, the tree, the grass,
the cloud, the sea, friend, enemy,
all of a kind, love.

Love is here, in silence,
in luminous darkness
before and beyond
the Beginning, the Big Bang,
the Word made flesh,
even Interdependent Arising.

Each step in the labyrinth,
each flash across the sky
and the enfolding brain,
connects us in one embrace.

Forget your fine distinctions,
the so-called conflicts,

the judgments on the types of love:
agape, eros, philia, storge,
metta, and all the rest —
all arise and bless each other
now and in the long run.

Shiva and David's dances,
Sarah's laugh and Hagar's tears,
become Lao-Tzu's flow,
the Buddha's flower, Kuan-Yin's kiss,
round of Jesus-Marys-Johns-Thomas-
Francis-Clare and their fond fools,
Cordelia's last breath apparent,
whirl of Sufis, Yaqui deer-dance,
followers of the drinking gourd,
and children spinning themselves
dizzy on a broken sidewalk.

Healing beyond healing,
embrace before embrace.
We come and go,
somehow we know
Love holds and moves us still.

— John Clarke

Forgiveness... The Gift You Give Yourself

by Julia B. Riley

HAVE YOU EVER HEARD a single sentence that changed your life? In 1999, at Omega Institute in Rhinebeck, New York, at a week-long Spiritual Eldering workshop, I heard Rabbi Zalman Schachter-Shalomi introduce the concept of forgiveness by saying, "Not forgiving someone is like stabbing yourself in the stomach to hurt the person standing behind you." What could this mean? What about righteous indignation? What about "unforgiveable" transgressions? What would it mean to forgive? Would that mean condoning the act? This began my ongoing journey to understand, practice, and facilitate the process of forgiveness.

Why forgive and how to forgive is the topic of this article. The tools and processes it explores draw on three sources: the work of Sage-ing (originally called Spiritual Eldering); research at the International Forgiveness Institute (which is the outgrowth of the social scientific research done at the University of Wisconsin-Madison since 1985 by Robert Enright and his colleagues); and one of Enright's books, *Forgiveness Is a Choice*.[1]

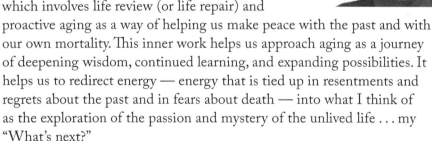

Sage-ing is an approach to conscious aging which involves life review (or life repair) and proactive aging as a way of helping us make peace with the past and with our own mortality. This inner work helps us approach aging as a journey of deepening wisdom, continued learning, and expanding possibilities. It helps us to redirect energy — energy that is tied up in resentments and regrets about the past and in fears about death — into what I think of as the exploration of the passion and mystery of the unlived life ... my "What's next?"

As we age we may dwell on the past, focusing on what we see as mistakes, missed opportunities, roads not taken. When we feel consumed by the resulting anxiety, we often take refuge in distracting activities to ward off the painful memories. A friend who has an issue with weight control says, "A sandwich is my friend." Reb Zalman writes that as we become determined to overcome this anxiety and remain present to the pain of past experiences, we discover to our surprise that the pain is eminently workable, that we can forgive ourselves. By befriending the pain, gently reviewing our past with the blessing of the wisdom gleaned in our lives, we can mend our personal history.

Time is stretchable and therefore subject to reshaping by contemplative techniques. One such process is called "Healing a Painful Memory," in which one reaches back into the past to heal the part of ourselves that is still imprisoned there — a questionable decision, a bruised relationship — and apply the balm of our more mature consciousness. In such a process we can see our elder self saying, "I come with assurance from the future. You are going to make it. You lived through this difficulty, healed from it, and learned important lessons that matured into wisdom."

To make peace with the past we must learn to forgive. Sage-ing offers two other processes I've found helpful in this regard:

> "A Testimonial Dinner for Life's Severe Teachers"[2] uses the broad perspective of time to "reframe" hurtful relationships and situations. You identify the lessons learned in an imagery or journal exercise; examine your own role, if any, in a given situation; consider the personal growth or good that might have come from the situation; forgive yourself if you had a part in causing the hurt; and then forgive the other, releasing the energy that has been tied up in resentment, and redirecting that energy into your conscious growth as an elder. For me, having had troubled relationships with my father and mother, I now acknowledge the gifts they have brought to my life, my father's gift of public speaking and my mother's joyful, playful outgoing personality... traits that have served me well.
>
> The second exercise — "Bedtime Prayer of Forgiveness" — is a preventive that uses simple contemplation before sleep to let go of and forgive transgressions of the day. I combine this with a nightly gratitude practice,[3] deep breaths of release, and a few moments to count my blessings. Emmons' research on the health benefits of a gratitude practice makes sense to me as a nurse. Here is a poem that captures the essence of this work:

The Sage Must Travel Light

Youth can carry a heavy load day after day
Without noticing the damaging effects,
But the sage must lay down the burden.
Resentments, regrets, injuries, slights,
Grudges and disappointments,
Are much too cumbersome
For a person of wisdom and contentment.
The sage must travel light.
There is a backpack in the mind
Which over the years has become
Filled with rock and stones.
You do not have to carry them anymore.
You can empty your pack
And carry only compassion from one day to the next.
— William Martin[4]

During my early research in 2000, I had come upon the home page of the International Forgiveness Institute, and there I found useful definitions that were starting points for my own thinking. Forgiveness IS a turning to the "good" in the face of wrongdoing, a foregoing of resentment or revenge even when it is deserved, a gift we give ourselves. Forgiveness IS NOT forgetting, denying, condoning, or seeking justice or compensation. Nor is forgiveness a quid-pro-quo exchange that seeks advanced compensation before its conferring.

In researching this article, I revisited the Institute, delving more deeply into the research by Robert Enright at the heart of their outreach. Forgiveness is clearly a skill that improves with practice; yet, more than a skill, it is an *attitude* of good will and a "moral virtue" that develops. It becomes a part of your identity and transforms your character and relationships as you understand and practice it. Not a quick fix — hard, sometimes painful — Enright likens his process to a road map that is checked for directions as needed.

Why do this? To get the pain to stop, to heal, and move on. He identifies the paradox of forgiving, that as we forgive the other who hurt us, we are the ones healed. *How to do this?* Enright's four steps or "guideposts" for forgiving include:

- uncovering your anger — anger can be a good motivator;

- deciding to forgive — creating a change of heart with a decision to forgive;

- working on forgiveness — to "begin to bear and grieve the pain" (Reed);

- releasing yourself from an emotional prison — and thereby perhaps finding meaning or even a new or renewed purpose in life.

This process involves using a journal as a guide to help you answer specific questions. The research that supports this work is impressive. Dr. Gayle Reed, who is also a personal counselor with Forgiveness Recovery, LLC, described how "research from the University of Wisconsin has shown that internalizing, or holding on to, hurt and resentment can lead to depression, post-traumatic stress, increased anger, anxiety, illness, drug and alcohol abuse, sleep- and even eating disorders. But the challenge is that simply saying 'I forgive you' isn't enough. True healing can come only when a person has committed to the process of forgiving."[5]

Waltman and colleagues did some compelling research on the effects of forgiveness on coronary artery disease. Their work provided a groundbreaking demonstration that health may be improved by an intervention that helps people to forgive someone who has caused them ongoing stress and grief.[6] They used myocardial perfusion imaging to show that vividly recalling a time when the patient was hurt by someone resulted in less disruption of their cardiac blood flow after 10 sessions of the forgiveness intervention, whereas 10 sessions of learning positive coping strategies did not improve blood flow. Theory would predict that the effect of the forgiveness intervention should be mediated by increased forgiveness and decreased anger, and these were indeed observed in the intervention group to a greater extent than in the control group.

If forgiveness is a skill that can be learned with practice, how might we introduce it to the children in our lives so that it becomes a lifelong skill? As a psychiatric nurse I wanted to help my son and myself to move through rough spots, to let go of anger and hurts, yet honor the power of the feelings. When we had a disagreement and I identified a time when it seemed we could move on, I would ask him, "Are you ready to start over?"

This meant lovingly letting go and moving on, with the understanding that he could refuse if he needed more time. It worked both ways as he got older. This seemed to clear the air. Enright has written a children's book to help a child imagine what forgiveness might look like... "getting in the plane, taking off, and rising above the story until you are bouncing gently on big white cotton ball clouds with the blue sky and sun ahead of you all day. Think of forgiveness this way."[7] I will offer this book to my grandchildren.

HAVE YOU EVER HEARD a single sentence that changed your life? Still learning... Several weeks ago I read a simple prayer, "Oh, Lord, please help me to forgive those who sin differently than I do." I continue to embrace "pithy prose" on life's journey of offering forgiveness to others and to myself. Forgiveness is a precious gift you give yourself.

In *The Second Half of Life: Opening the Eight Gates of Wisdom*, Angeles Arrien guides the reader through "metaphorical gates of initiation" — gates she says we must each pass through if we hope to become fully actualized elders. Her "archetypal passageways" map a new landscape for the second half of life richly grounded in multicultural traditions that honor elders. For each gate, Arrien offers a task, challenge, gift, reflections, and practice. Poignant images of hands and feet set off each chapter, and poems and inspirational quotes add to the fullness. This profound, beautiful book provided an awakening and spiritual itinerary that enabled me in my early fifties to shift my perspective and embrace the aging process. I return to it often for inspiration — each gate is experienced differently from one year or decade to the next, and the book's riches are revealed anew with each reading.

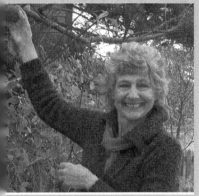

Deborah Windrum

    Deborah F. Windrum, independent author/presenter and librarian at the University of Colorado Boulder, wrote *Harvest the Bounty of Your Career* in order to reconcile the persistent demands of a career with evolving priorities in the second half of life. Harvest is about appreciating the natural cycles of life's seasons, distilling the gifts of work, and cultivating a new season of life.

Honoring the Cycles of Our Inner Seasons

by Deborah Windrum

Do you remember being asked as a child: *What do you want to be when you grow up?* What image did this question generate? Dressing in a white coat and stethoscope to provide care? Writing on a chalkboard to teach? Performing athletic feats? Protecting the innocent and punishing the guilty? Making music or art? Nurturing your own children? Your response probably stimulated your imagination and planted seeds of possibilities. Many of us find that one or more of those seeds do take root, and over time we embrace the qualities of the roles we imagined as children.

As youthful adults, we busily till, plant, and cultivate the landscape of our lives. We are the architect of our dreams, goals, education, work, family, and material needs and wants. We choose what to do, and we are asked: *How are you doing?* Over time, we notice how we *feel* in the doing.

And then how quickly the landscape of life reaches full bloom, and the weather begins to change, suggesting the onset of a new season, new priorities. Interest in retiring from employment may arise when our preoccupation with the outer landscape gives way to a desire to create greater balance in our lives. "The actual task is to integrate the two threads of one's life," the French philosopher and Jesuit priest, Pierre Teilhard de Chardin, wrote, "the within and the without." The inner landscape and the relationship between the inner and the outer become as compelling as being busy in the world.

The usual question at this transition point is, "What do you want to do when you retire?" And the most frequent response, according to Tammy Erickson, expert on workforce and demographic trends, is "Take a cruise." After decades of employment, most of us would benefit from a break and a significant transitional event. However, the most important question is not *What will you DO?* in retirement or your second half of life or your third age. The question is not even: *What do you want to be when you retire?* The question is: *How will you be?* And then: *How are you being?*

Doing and being, of course, are not polarities and cannot be separated. Doing is about activities, and quantity counts. Being is the degree of awareness manifested, whether the activity is bicycling, computing, or meditating. We all know the difference between being hyperfocused, distracted, or fully present. When we attend to the quality of our being, the what and how of doing simply flow. This is the developmental possibility of life's autumn season.

Each season or stage of life offers opportunities to cultivate personal growth. For the infant, growth must be supported by caretakers. Throughout youth, developmental markers that bring us to independence are celebrated. Despite the coincident doubts, confusion, and heartbreak, many grownups never stop yearning for youth's aliveness, beauty, and promise. But obsession with youth has created an "ever-summer" culture, in which people forever explore the adolescent fascination with sex and violence — bastions of Hollywood and network television.

A never-ending summer requires the denial of winter and diminishes the developmental benefits of appropriately timed spring and autumn seasons. The sweetness and slowness of childhood's spring are sacrificed in the rush to summer; preadolescent girls dress for sex appeal earlier and earlier, while boys experiment with danger at younger and younger ages. The gradual process of development that extends the magic of childhood into the teens is arrested.

No less important than an appropriate springtime of life, an autumn season is the developmental stage that brings us to true maturity. It need not be the staid, boring, narrow maturity which we once repudiated in those over 30. We can choose a ripeness of being that is expansive, creative, embracing, accepting. Baby Boomers are now learning that an extended transitional period is important to make a shift from working for a living to living a next life stage. Most of us who have been actively employed for decades are not likely to be suddenly comfortable with a "restful" leisure that does not include meaningful social interaction and activities.

Fulfillment of each adult life stage is more likely when it is preceded by a period of conscious transition. And our extended life span offers the opportunity to transition effectively into our autumn and winter seasons. Winter, especially, is more likely to provide fulfillment when it follows a developmentally healthy and satisfying autumn. The fact that winter's life-giving importance lies beneath the surface makes it no less vital and purposeful; winter is the final stage of growth that allows us to become fully who we are. As James Hillman says, in *The Force of Character and the Lasting Life*: "Aging is no accident. It is necessary to the human condition, intended by the soul. We become more characteristic of who we are simply by lasting into later years; the older we become, the more our true natures emerge. Thus the final years have a very important purpose: the fulfillment and confirmation of one's character."

Aging is, in fact, very attractive to me about now. At 61, I'm one year into my seventh decade. I'm also a full-time librarian in an understaffed, underfunded, and nevertheless striving and thriving academic library. As a professional, I remain busy beyond a newly developing comfort zone. Although, given the fact that U.S. productivity grew by over 60 per cent between 1989 to 2010, it may be that my stamina is challenged due to not only my increasing age, but also expanding expectations of increasing performance with diminishing monetary compensation.

Whatever the complex of conditions, I find myself in the autumn of my life as overloaded as my younger colleagues and filled, not with their befitting ambition to achieve, but with longing for some of the enticements of age — more time for contemplation, more expansiveness, more space for evolving priorities. Despite the media's offerings of lasting youth, I am not interested in staying young or getting younger.

I am, however, interested in "youthfulness," as well as "agefulness." Both youthful and ageful are qualities of being. And one of the pleasures of aging is that, while we continue to enjoy qualities that serve us, we also are positioned to consciously choose and develop qualities that may have eluded our younger selves, including those inherent in vocations that appealed to us as youngsters.

The autumn season offers an opportunity to create a deliberate blueprint for living — to notice how we want to be in order to choose what we want to do. With the advantages of youth and adulthood — experiences, skills, knowledge, and acquired wisdom — we are positioned to become the considered architects of our beings. With qualities of agefulness, we have the opportunity to mindfully, consciously fulfill life's cycles — to embrace the heart of aging.

As I find myself feeling urged from within to enter into a more "age-appropriate" period in my life, it occurs to me that aging can be viewed as a "practice." There are at least two reasons to practice. When we practice to get better at something — a musical instrument, sport, or skill — we do so to *acquire* mastery of something. There is also practice that one integrates into life, such as yoga or meditation, not just to do, but also in order to be masterful in life.

A Practice of Aging

So, how do we make a practice of aging? How do we integrate such practice into our autumn season, which often seems to hold as much busy-ness as ever? How do we build a practice that does not require lengthy or consistent chunks of time or even a foreseeable conclusion?

Here is an exercise that can be embraced without adding any weight or pressure to your life. In fact, you may find that it lightens stress and energizes your sense of purpose:

Consider what qualities of youth and age you most appreciate. What traits do you admire in others? Which of your own attributes represent your best? What do you consider indicators of fulfillment? Allow the qualities you value to coalesce into an image or a sensation. A personified image may be based on a projection of yourself, an idealization of a real-life person, or someone completely imagined. A felt sensation may be represented with an abstract image, such as a symbol, graphic, shape, or color.

You may wish to collect pictures, or, even better, draw, color, paint, collage, sculpt, or otherwise manifest your image. Whenever you desire to soothe, reassure, or inspire yourself, experience the feelings evoked by your image. Notice and embrace each sign of aging as movement towards that image, and celebrate your progress. Claim and cultivate those feelings — they are the self-fulfilling blueprint of your ageful inner landscape.

A favorite colleague of mine, 42-year-old Andrew Violet, has long held an endearing image of himself as a wise, old man practicing yoga. Andrew finds it grounding to return to his yoga mat daily, and he believes the sense of groundedness will become amplified as he sustains the practice throughout his future. He calls it "simultaneity of timeline" as he joins his ageful self on the mat now. His image of the future yoga practitioner is his blueprint for aging.

My blueprint for agefulness derives from my maternal grandmother. Although she died when I was a young teen, I remember vividly the look and feel of her sweet, calm presence and her unconditional love for every family member. A revered matriarch, bonding the family together with her wisdom and warmth, clarity and strength, she was the steward of family traditions and provider of holiday feasts. (And, it doesn't matter at all for my practice whether my memories are based on accurate perceptions or childish idealism.)

My heart's depiction of my grandmother is my blueprint for agefulness. Every time I appreciate her qualities, I strengthen those same qualities within myself. Every time I savor the sweetness of her image, I embrace my own progress towards that future landscape. The traits she personifies are my vows to self, as I repeat the mantra that "I am the seed of her seed; she is a seed in me."

Are you ready and willing to transition from summer without artificially prolonging the season? Will you embrace life's autumn to experience it fully? Will you hold an image of agefulness now, practicing so that you will "become of age" in the wisdom of your winter season? *That* is aging in practice.

Sugaring

Tapping the trees of memories
boiling down the sap
of long and challenging years,
siphoning off old sorrows and the dross,
I gather at last
that sweet syrup of life!

— Helen Vanier[†]

[†] Published in *Celebrating Poets over 70*, M. Vespry and E. Ryan, editors (McMaster Centre for Gerontological Studies, 2010).

I am that old lady now

I hear myself
talking to me,
sometimes in a whisper
sometimes out loud.
I smile —
How often I teased
my grandma
for her soft
soliloquies.

I try to do it softly,
unwrapping my mint
in church;
I don't want to
irritate the young ones
like those old women
irritated me.

I cannot always find
that precise word
that I need —
So lucky my girls
are too far away
to tease me
the way I did my mum.

I look in the mirror
and see my snow white hair,
And again I smile —
I did not become
one of those
blue-haired ladies
after all!
  — Desiré Lyners Volkwijn

The Epiphany of Life-Altering Illnesses

by Louden Kiracofe

IN 1912 JAPAN SENT MORE than 3,000 cherry trees to America as a gift of friendship. Most were planted around the Tidal Basin in Washington, DC. They bloom every year and are at their peak in early April. Tens of thousands of visitors come to see this magnificent and transient show of beauty. If the trees were in full blossom throughout the year, we would not be so deeply awed by their splendor nor would so many travel so far to view their display. Their beauty would be taken for granted. But the show is transient. As such, it can be symbolic of our mortality. If we lived forever, each day would lose the quality of the remarkably wonderful and sacred gift of life that it truly is. It is this background of mortality that reminds us how precious life is. Yet, mortality becomes a concept rather than a reality for most of us. And so we forget the miracle of being alive. We take it for granted.

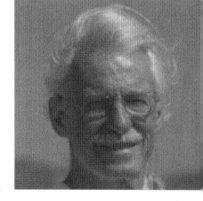

Over the past many years, I've had the privilege of being a facilitator of support groups for people who are suddenly confronted with life-altering illnesses. I have often seen the multidimensional dynamics that unfold when we are informed by our physician that we have cancer, serious heart disease, or that a risky surgical procedure is required for a newly diagnosed problem. Initially, the impact of this announcement may well result in fear, anger, and depression. As we move through the complex medical procedures that we often must endure to establish the diagnosis, plan a treatment strategy, and become immersed in that treatment, we may feel helpless, without hope, and dehumanized.

Modern medicine, solidly based in the scientific paradigm, has made incredible advances in surgical techniques, e.g., robotic and laser surgical procedures. The results of chemotherapy for some cancers have worked near-miraculous cures. New drugs are on the near horizon that may well establish genetic manipulation as a common treatment for some illnesses that are currently incurable. Yet this medical paradigm concentrates almost exclusively on *quantity* rather than *quality* of life. Its objective is to cure the problem as quickly and efficiently as possible and to return us to "normal" life as soon as possible. Little to no consideration is given to the impact of the illness upon the psychosocial and spiritual dimensions of our lives.

Our medical model is focused on *cures* and not on the much broader reality connoted by the word *healing*.

It is important that we remember that health is much more than physical well-being. We all know people who, after extensive tests and rigorous physical examinations, are declared in "perfect" health. Yet these very same people may be suffering from severe stress, toxic personal relationships, poor self image, or deadening work. In the broader sense of health, these people are not healthy!

Along with the fear, anger, and despair that are commonly experienced when we find that we are faced with a life-altering illness, there can also be a dramatic shift in our priorities. The amount of money in our account, that new car we were hoping to purchase, plans for renovating the home — all these "things" become secondary. Our attention is shifted to relationships, to our spiritual life, to the importance of being alive and enjoying this very day which we suddenly realize is a wonderful gift that comes with no guarantees for yet another. We are mortal after all! I have known many people with severe chronic diseases, such as diabetes, heart disease, life-restricting pulmonary problems, and even cancer, who, nevertheless, are living happy and productive lives. They are enjoying loving relationships, meaningful friendships, are involved in occupations or projects that are deeply rewarding, and doing so with the knowledge that their remaining life may be limited to months or weeks. Physical health is a means to an end and not an end in itself!

We all come into this world as unique persons. And we all have in common certain important needs: to love and to be loved; to touch and be touched; to be happy in our relationships with loved ones and friends who will see us, hear us, and honor our presence in their lives. Still, no two of us are exactly alike. And in our differences lies a special gift that each of us brings, a quality that defines more than any other who we are. This gift can be easily lost in the course of our efforts to "fit in," to "be accepted" by family and peers, and to achieve the goals that our culture deems important. Yet, this gift must be manifested in our lives if we are to be truly happy, fulfilled, and at peace. Two stories exemplify this well:

A dear friend was found several years ago to have multiple myeloma, a bone cancer that, even with aggressive treatment, usually results in only a 30 to 40 percent survival five years after the diagnosis is made. As his illness steady progressed, his focus upon and complete appreciation and enjoyment of each day as a special gift progressed as well. He knew his time was very limited, and he spent as much of it as possible with his friends and made a host of new ones. He accepted with gratitude the love and help he was offered and threw himself fully into the completion of a history book that he had been working on from time to time for the past 20-plus years. He lived to see his book published and to sign a copy and place it in my hands. And even in the hardest of times he felt a peacefulness that came from being fully committed to living one day at a time. He exemplified the quality of life that a person can have when they listen with open hearts to the message of a life-altering illness. Investing one's self fully into this very day, allowing neither the fears and anxieties of tomorrow nor the anger and guilt of yesterday to intrude, we can joyfully accept each moment as a precious gift. This shift in our attitude is transformational for us and all those around us.

A colleague, Jim, was a successful and very busy cardiologist. He was involved in a program for heart disease prevention that included a group support meeting. He decided to "sit in" on a meeting and was so moved by the personal stories of the participants that he continued to come to the meetings as a participant himself. He realized that he'd become an excellent doctor of illness, but had abandoned his initial dream of being a healer of people. He began to develop personal relationships with his patients which he said added perhaps an additional five minutes to an office visit, but the return was a richer and more rewarding practice experience. He returned to his initial goal and his gift of caring for people, and was happier in his work than ever before.

When the "wake-up call" of our mortality comes, our attention can shift dramatically. As we age, such "wake-ups" are more frequent. It need not be a diagnosis of cancer. It can be the loss of a close friend or a significant illness in a loved one. It can even be the gradual and inevitable loss of our physical abilities: having to have a knee replacement, giving up tennis because of arthritis in our shoulder, the slowing of our mental faculties. It is never too late to hear the message of our mortality. Rather than ignoring this message and trying to escape from its reality by diving even deeper into the work and ambitions that have not brought us real happiness, we can seek within the discomfort of these events the *voice* of the illness that says, "You really are mortal! Now is the time to pay attention to what is really important! You don't have time to squander on such foolishness as anger, spitefulness, and grudges, or to remain unforgiving of yourself and others." When we can hear this, we can begin to focus on healing relationships, allowing ourselves to love and be loved, really appreciating the glory of one more day of life as a precious gift, even when, or especially when, we realize that the prospect for longevity is improbable.

When initially diagnosed, Tony already had advanced cancer which had spread to his bones. As a child from a poor family, in a gang-infested part of Denver, he had been abandoned by his father and suffered physical abuse from his brothers and their friends. He had searched for his father most of his life with no success. In spite of these problems, he had risen to become an executive for a major national news service. But he had become chronically angry and had learned to protect himself by shutting himself off from any emotional access. He refused to open his heart to the love of a woman who was caring for him. During the course of coming to terms with his illness, he realized he had pushed away others and made himself a lonely and isolated man. He decided to allow this woman's love in. It took courage and faith to do so, but the result was a happiness he'd never experienced before and which brought joy and meaning into the last years of his life. In a talk I was giving to our local medical staff about the importance of support groups for people with life-altering illnesses, I asked if there were any comments. Tony stood and said, "Thank God for cancer! It opened my eyes to what was missing in my life and gave me the courage to open my heart!"

Bob was a member of our support group. He had been found to have prostate cancer and had undergone an operation that had apparently resulted in a total cure. There was no evidence of any lingering or recurrent malignancy. But from his experience he had learned that his priorities were not in harmony with the more important desires of his life. He had drifted apart from a brother and hadn't spoken to him for years. He announced one evening in our meeting that he was going to call him even though he didn't know whether his call would be appreciated or not. He was going to make contact anyway. He came to the next meeting full of joy. His brother was delighted to have heard from him, and they were planning a reunion. A simple but courageous and mindful act brought great joy into the lives of two people. And it may never have occurred had it not been for Bob's ability to listen to the "message" of his experience with illness.

The cherry tree is still in bloom. Its transient beauty calls for us to turn away from the unimportant and fully indulge ourselves in its loveliness — to be present right now! — and to revel in the splendor of *this* day.

Artistic Creativity As Renewal in Eldering

by Richard Matzkin

CREATIVE EXPRESSION IS AN ESSENTIAL aspect of the human spirit. In every place on the globe, in every era from prehistoric times to the present, humans have engaged in the creative arts.

The active aspects of artistic creativity involve an individual taking that which is free to be molded — be it art materials, musical notes, written words, vocalization, or body movement — and manipulating it in a way that becomes a personal expression. Its counterpart is passive appreciation, which also demands creativity. Just as creating art can evoke thought and feeling in the one creating it, experiencing that art — listening to or watching a performance, or viewing an art piece — can also evoke thought and feeling in the participant.

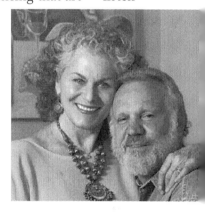

Much has been written about the power of the arts to heal. More recently, with the graying of our population, there has been a shift of focus onto elders. Research has shown that while certain aspects of brain function decline with age, such as short-term memory, speed of recall, and reaction time, creativity can remain relatively untouched and flourish throughout the life cycle.

In a landmark study by the late Gene Cohen, elders who engaged in group participatory visual art programs (average age 80) exhibited general improvement in physical and mental health, including reduced medication and fewer doctor visits. A study by the Medical School of New York University found that Alzheimer's patients exhibited fewer problems, increased self-esteem, elevated mood, and improved social interaction following visits to art museums.

My own experience as a sculptor and jazz musician provides a hint as to what might be occurring during the creative act that would account for these healing effects. As I engage in sculpting or playing music, I enter an altered state of consciousness akin to meditation. My discursive mind turns off or fades into the background; I am not aware of my body; time ceases to exist; there is no past, no future, only the present moment. All that exists is fingers moving clay or the flow of the music.

One doesn't have to be a professional artist, musical genius, or Zen master to enter this flow. My wife, Alice, a painter, and I have conducted beginner's art workshops for adults at community colleges, taught art to children, and worked using art therapy in psychiatric hospitals. Almost invariably, as a roomful of people become absorbed in their work, the silence and the sense of peace in the room are palpable.

The act of creation is a living, breathing process. You are giving birth to something from deep inside yourself — your unique expression. Creating a piece of art presents you with the opportunity to proclaim, "This may not be a masterpiece, but this is who I am … This is what I have created!" This can be especially satisfying and empowering for elders, who see their sense of control and authority gradually slip away as they age and become less "productive."

Another factor that makes creative work so engrossing is the element of surprise, of improvisation. As the composer composes, the artist paints, the poet writes, each note, each brush stroke, each word is an exploration that carries the artist along into the unknown. I watched a film, shot over a period of several days, of Picasso painting a portrait. In that time the painting went through numerous transformations before Picasso finally brought it to completion. This element of exploration, of stepping into the unknown, is the very essence of creativity, and it is the antithesis of stagnation. Stagnation — being bored, listless, uninvolved — can be a plague of the elder years, when the weight of disability or a "been there, done that" attitude can dampen one's vitality. Stagnation is as deadly as any disease.

Artistic creation has played an important role in my renewal and also that of my wife, Alice. Both of us possessed artistic gifts as we were growing up — skills which lay fallow as we were raising children and pursuing careers. In our 40s, our creative fires were rekindled and we returned to painting and sculpting. As we entered our 50s and felt the physical effects of aging, we began to use our art as a way to explore our issues about growing old and dying. Thus began a series of projects related to aging that brought our fears and anxieties to the surface where they could be consciously experienced, worked through, and transformed into understanding. Those projects — portraits of inspiring elder women; sculptures of old men in dissolution; paintings of elder nude women; sculptures of old couples in tender embrace; and sequential portraits of an aunt ages 89–97, showing the progressive effects of age on the body — helped us come to a deeper acceptance of and understanding about our own process of aging, and led us to value the preciousness of each present moment.

In time, we were able to add another medium to our creative arsenal, writing. Inspired by the focus that our artwork brought, we authored an award-winning book, *The Art of Aging: Celebrating the Authentic Aging Self*. With speaking engagements and additional projects, we find ourselves today, at ages 68 and 71, busier, more creative, and more engaged than at any other period in our lives.

Age is no barrier to creativity. Examples abound of elder artists whose creative production extends into late old age. Our neighbor, the potter Beatrice Wood, continued drawing and throwing pots until she was 105 years old. The autumn and winter of life is an optimum time for engaging in creative activity. Retirement and liberation from child rearing allows leisure time for exploration into creative resources. Elders have more life experience to draw upon to fuel artistic endeavors. Wisdom, wider perspective, and maturity of years lived can allow creativity to blossom with greater depth and richness. And that creative juice can invigorate the body, vitalize the mind, and renew the spirit in our elder years.

The Day Dad Died

Someone making coffee, lists,
    phone calls.

Yesterday's completed crossword puzzle
beside library books marked in progress;
jars of crab apple jelly on the counter,
    varied hues of first-time experimenting.

Garden grey in November bleak,
plants shrunken into earth, yet
on the anniversary rosebush, barren all summer,
    two yellow blooms.
                        — Ellen B. Ryan

Now I Notice Sea Shells

Age ten I charge surf at high tide
leap with thunder and roll
hours in swarming-cousins heat
Set aglide by curl of longed-for wave
I yearn for next year stronger, faster
Conch shell calls, horizon beckons

Age sixty I wade along low-tide beach
pants rolled up, jacketed for off-season cool
Seagulls and sandpipers scurry ahead
Pelicans swoop, sunset shadows stretch
colours shifting as sky reflections ebb
Conch shell woos me deep inside
                        — Ellen B. Ryan

Invitations to Practice

Fierce with Age:
The Opening Exercise

by Carol Orsborn

In answering the call to help others confront, face, and transcend the stereotypes of aging, I developed a retreat that I now take into churches, the aging community, and healthcare organizations. The retreat, which is also available in an online version, begins with a "wake-up" exercise. In this opening exercise, I begin by asking participants to consider their judgments of individuals their age and older. Here's the exercise, for you to follow along.

So who do you think is an example of someone who is aging well — and someone who is aging badly? What I'd like you to do is make a separate list of characteristics for each of your examples. What adjectives, qualities, and characteristics best describe the essence of the individual you chose as someone who is aging well? On a separate list, what adjectives, qualities, and characteristics best describe the essence of the individual you chose who is aging badly?

The essence of this first lesson is this: The lists you came up with say as much about you as they do about the person you selected. The list that describes someone who is aging well gives you a vivid, concrete profile of the aspirations you hold in regards to aging. Not every adjective you put on the list may apply to you, but the list — as a whole — will provide you with interesting insights about yourself. The list that described someone who is aging badly also provides you with insight, but in this case you are provided a portal into what it is you most fear about aging: your concerns and your issues.

For the purposes of this exercise as an illustration of what it means to become fierce with age, we are going to be concentrating on mining the wisdom from your list of attributes for the individual who is aging well. So begin by taking a look at the list of adjectives, qualities, and characteristics you used to describe the individual who is aging well. To mine the lesson from this assignment, go ahead and circle every item on the list that is NOT necessarily dependent on one's circumstances. As you circle the items that are not dependent on circumstances, keep in mind that the items you choose to circle will often require a judgment call on your part. For instance, we can probably agree that a person can have a great sense of humor more or less regardless of whatever else is going on in their lives. If you agree, you would go ahead and circle "great sense of humor." Items like "resilient" and "has an optimistic attitude" would fall into this category.

Now let's take another example: "Has a great job." Having a great job is not always a matter of personal control. People get laid off or retire, companies merge, individuals develop a disability. Yes, we can do whatever we can to keep our jobs or make ourselves as employable as possible, but we cannot guarantee that we will have great jobs for the rest of our lives. I would suggest that you not circle this item.

How about "healthy" or "athletic"? Yes, we can influence our health and level of physical fitness — but we cannot guarantee that we will never develop an ailment or face some manner of physical challenge down the road. I would suggest that you NOT circle "healthy" or any of its variations. If you are confused or conflicted about any particular item, don't circle it.

What you are left with is two buckets. In the first bucket are all the circled items: items that you admire and that you are clear are under your control to cultivate in yourself, regardless of the circumstances of your life now and down the road. In the second bucket are all the uncircled items that are certainly or potentially dependent on circumstances beyond your control.

Knowledge is power. Your original list provides you with a vivid and concrete picture of your aspirations for the future. Chances are you will have the good fortune of aging as graciously as the individual whom you have identified as aging well. You are way ahead of the game, knowing what it is you would like for yourself and using this as a spur to do whatever you can to make this vision your reality. But here's something important to think about. The more uncircled items there are on your list, the more likely you are to be feeling unsettled about the future. If this is the case, it is because on some level you already suspect that you are placing faith in that which is ultimately undependable. Of course we should do whatever we can within our power to influence the circumstances of our lives, but there is a cost to denying that our power is limited. The good news is that once we break denial, we gain immediate access to the entire range of our abundant internal as well as external resources, to begin to build a spiritually and psychologically healthy vision of aging that can be counted upon to go the distance.

Key Take-Away Message

A key take-away from this first exercise — and the foundation of the discipline of viewing aging as a spiritual practice — is that those of us who can grow large enough to embrace rather than deny the shadow side of aging can organically have what the eastern traditions call an "awakening." We don't need books to help us understand the transitory nature of life. We are living it.

If this were all there were to it, however, we'd all be mystics basking on the river bank of old age. We all know, however, that getting older does not necessarily guarantee spiritual attainment, wisdom, or even peace. Who hasn't encountered bitter, cynical, or resigned individuals who see aging only in terms of what is being taken away from them? As I said earlier, the truth is that the aging process requires a level of ongoing spiritual commitment that is a challenge to the best of us.

By continuing to immerse myself in the conscious aging literature, practice, ritual, and conversation, most if not all the negative connotations of being old have dropped away for me. I have stopped seeing age as illness and imposition, and have begun seeing it as increased freedom and activation of new, unprecedented levels of self-affirmation and spiritual growth. So now, when I say "I'm old," this represents the overthrowing of the stereotypes and the reclamation of the integrity of the fullness of life I now see as my God-given right. In fact, I am excited about exploring this new stage of life. This initiation of a fresh life stage bears with it the hallmarks of all the previous life stages combined: the high anticipation, the celebration, and the bold, outright terror. In other words, aging has become transformed into a spiritual path, not only a continuation but an acceleration of the journey towards fulfillment of the true human potential.

As I conclude in my memoir: "Plummet into aging, stare mortality in the eye, surrender everything and what else is there left to fear? The way is perilous, danger on all sides. But we can be part of a generation no longer afraid of age. We are becoming, instead, a generation fierce with age."[†]

[†] Carol Orsborn, *Fierce with Age: Chasing God and Squirrels in Brooklyn* (Turner Publishing Company, 2013).

Part II

Aging as a Spiritual Practice

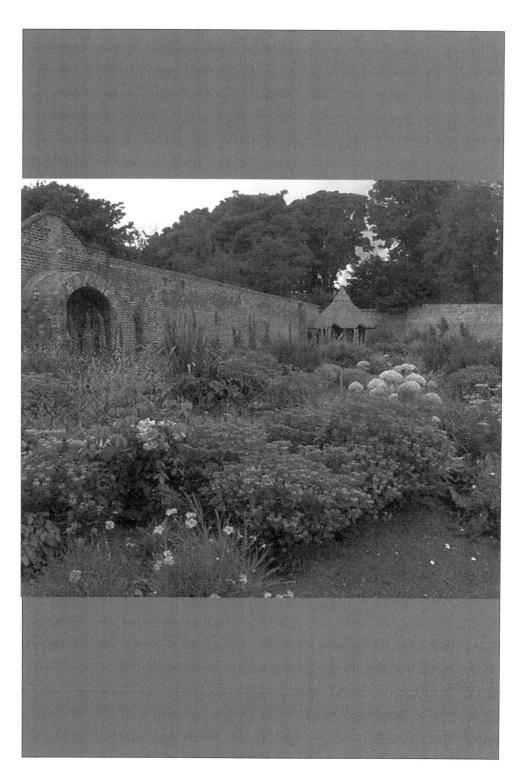

Excavations: A Life in Three Parts

by Bolton Anthony

The great reward from mining our life experience comes when we strike that *vein of purpose* and find that the seemingly diffused endeavors and commitments of our life cohere. A hidden pattern is revealed, a "strange attractor" around which the once random trajectories of our life now constellate, disclosed. And we arrive at the place where "everything belongs" — ready, as the poet Yeats says, "to cast out remorse" and "live it all again and yet again."

Why did God make you? Every Catholic of a certain age — as part of their early catechetical drilling — will have been asked this sixth question from the *Baltimore Catechism* and been expected to answer: *God made me to know Him, to love Him, and to serve Him in this world, and to be happy with Him forever in heaven.* If the child took this teaching to heart, he stepped through a door and embarked on a quest to untangle the mysterious threads of purpose in his life.

Of the four parts of the answer, it was the third — perhaps because it seemed the only one I could *do* something about, the only area of action in my control — that ignited my passion. Like all great teaching, the "answer" is just a trove of further questions: *How* did I serve God in this world? What was my *calling*, my *vocation*? What was to be my work in the world?

But there was something too constricted in the way these questions came to be framed for me. For a life to be worth living, it had to be a life worth dying for. That became the test of authenticity. For the child that I was, enfolded by ritual, with a love for learning and a gift for writing, there seemed only three career paths that were legitimate: I could become a priest, a teacher, or a writer.

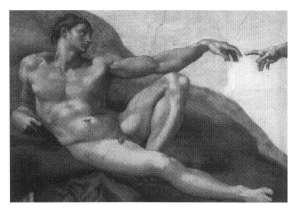

As I moved through my student years, then into my householding years, I found myself progressively barred from each of these paths. In puberty I discovered girls and ruled out a life of celibacy. I married, started a family, and embarked on making a living. I couldn't do it as a writer; my gift was perhaps too small, my dedication too tepid, or the demands on my time too many. So I became a teacher.

We were standing at the edge of the playground with the high fortress-like wall behind us. To be heard over the noise of the playing children, I had raised my voice. Tamping his hand down, my colleague cautioned me. He nodded imperceptibly, and I followed the direction of his nod to where an old hag of a nun was watching us from an open second-story window.
— The principal will hear you.
— And well she should, I said. I'll tell her what I think of how this place is run. Do you know what I'm doing these days… after I wander the hallways for an hour or two looking for my class? I come out and work in the garden, just to have something productive to do. No, let her come talk to me. In fact, I want to see the Registrar.

I finished a master's degree in creative writing and, in the fall of 1967, took my first job teaching English at Xavier University, a Black university in New Orleans. I was returning to the city of my birth after an absence of 16 years — returning at a strident and tumultuous moment in our history which, in my own life and the lives of my students, seemed to call into question the value of teaching and learning. Martin Luther King was shot during the spring of 1968, and Richard Nixon was elected the following fall.

I left Xavier the following year. Though I'd intended to pursue a doctorate at Notre Dame, where I'd been an undergraduate, I found immediately I couldn't afford that and instead ended up teaching part-time at several colleges near South Bend. I left teaching altogether three years later, after a final year at a prep school.

Though I pursued other career paths in my life — got a master's degree in Library Science and worked as a public librarian, got a doctorate in Educational Administration and worked as a university administrator — all these endeavors somehow seemed to come up short, to lack legitimacy, measured against the standards ingrained in childhood.

Excavations: A Life in Three Parts

The texts I have been inserting are the episodes from a dream — one of a number of powerful dreams I had the year I turned 50. It came as a blessing and a dispensation that what had seemed like no path was indeed a genuine path.

> I was using a hoe to weed the garden plot tucked into a corner where two high walls intersected, when I caught sight of him striding toward me across the wide lawn. He was a behemoth of a man, dressed in a clerical black suit that shimmered as the sun danced over it. He stopped when he drew close.
> — You asked to see the Registrar? Well, I am the Registrar.
> I minced no words telling him how poorly I thought the school was run. — I am a teacher, I said, and there are students here who need me.
> He ignored my diatribe as he surveyed my work. Then, looking at me, he said, — So these are the magnificent gardens everyone is talking about!
> I looked about me and saw the garden — lush and fragrant with flowering plants — as if for the first time. As we strolled the grounds together, he admiring the many landscaped areas we came across, I realized I had somehow managed to create all these beautiful inviting spaces, as it were, in my spare time. When we stopped at the end of our circuit, he looked at me.
> — You know, at our cloister in Montreal, I was a gardener too.

The dreams of my fiftieth year presaged tectonic shifts in my life. For the second time in five years, I was dealing with prolonged unemployment. My five children were raised, and the youngest would leave for college in the fall. My marriage of 28 years was dissolving. With hindsight I see that a demarcation line, between a first and second half of life, was being drawn. Within a fortnight of my "garden dream" I had moved out of our home in Greensboro, where I'd been living for 14 years, and taken a position at the University of North Carolina in Wilmington.

> In the dissolution of the partnership with Pugh in early 1862, [Darden] kept ownership of the St. Bernard [plantation which] with 600 argents, had had only 41 slaves (all listed by family), six

> cabins, a smaller sugarhouse valued at $4,500, a dwelling worth $1,500 and several lesser such structures.

Wilmington had had a troubled racial history, and the grant project I was hired to manage had as its focus race relations. I remember following the news coverage during the '70s of the Wilmington Ten, a group of civil rights activists who spent nearly a decade in jail for arson and conspiracy before the questionable verdict was overturned in 1980.

The 1971 incident could be thought of, however, as an aftershock of a much more gruesome secret buried in Wilmington's past. Wilmington near the turn of the last century had been the most populous city in the state and a magnet for aspiring Blacks who found opportunity in the city's building and shipping trades. Blacks made up 60 percent of

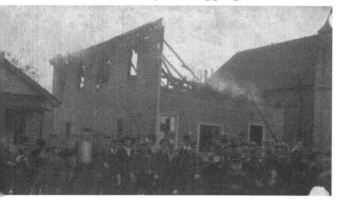

the population and held elected office on the City Council. On November 10, 1898, a white vigilante mob gathered before the offices of the state's only Black daily newspaper, the *Wilmington Daily Record*, to protest an editorial which the engaged white citizenry thought had defamed Southern womanhood. After burning down the building, then posing proudly for their photograph, the mob marched downtown; deposed the existing council and installed a rump one in its place; and issued a manifesto, its "Declaration of White Independence." For three days following, Republicans and Black entrepreneurs were put on trains leaving the city and told not to return. Estimates of the number of Black citizens who died in the violence go as high as 300. President William McKinley was kept fully informed of the events in this, the only instance of the illegal overthrow of a municipal government in U.S. history. He turned a blind eye.

When I arrived in Wilmington, the centennial anniversary of these tumultuous events was approaching. It took minimal investigative skills to see that dangerous memories[1] of the 1898 insurrection were poisoning race relations and needed to be exorcised in a way that only their solemn commemoration could accomplish. It was, however, an initiative that the university would not lead, sensitive as it had to be to political pressure; in a quirk of history, three key leaders of the 1898 conspiracy had living grandsons who bore their exact names and were prominent citizens in the community as well as current or former members of the university's Board of Trustees. In the end, I helped spearhead the creation of an independent foundation and served as its director as we planned, then implemented, a yearlong reconciliation effort.

There seemed to me that a great deal of chance played into my role in all of this. Hadn't I taken the temporary assignment in Wilmington simply as a last resort — the only available opening that offered the remotest chance of salvaging my battered resumé and maintaining some semblance of a career path that could lead to future employment? Hadn't I simply *fallen into* a leadership role — not so much an *outside* as an *accidental* agitator? Looking back now, however, a pattern is discernible. A passion for racial justice runs through my biography — a vein of purpose — from my first job teaching at a Black college to my work in Wilmington. I cannot trace its roots to conscious experiences: Though I grew up in the segregated South, we left New Orleans, where racial tensions simmered just below the surface, when I was six; and I grew up in Houston, insulated by my minority Catholic experience, from racism's rawest cultural expressions. If I could be said to have chosen this work, the part of me that did the choosing was deeper than ego and consciousness — some sort of bedrock self that knew exactly what it needed to do.

I'd been in Wilmington two years and was deeply involved with the centennial commemoration when I received an unexpected parcel from my mother. The pamphlet it contained — the early history of St. John's Episcopal Church in Thibodeaux, LA, written by the first pastor — gives brief biographies of the founding members of the vestry, including my great-great-grandfather, Richardson Gray Darden. The brief excerpt inserted earlier that describes the size of his plantation and the number of slaves he owned is taken from its text, as is the one below, which, when I first read it, sent quivers through me.

> Richardson Gray Darden was born on August 27, 1809, at Wilmington, North Carolina, one of 13 children of Reddick Darden and Catherine Thomas. [He and two of his brothers] joined the swelling migration of many citizens of that state to ... Deep South regions [including Louisiana, where he became] an overseer on sugar cane plantations.

There is a passage from the novel *A Flag for Sunrise* by Robert Stone where the revolutionary priest, Godoy, is described this way:

> He fights for the peasants and the Indians because whether he knows it or not, he *deeply desires the just rule of the Lord*. Probably, he will never realize this… But I think unconsciously it is the kingdom of God he fights for.[2]

I have a visceral memory of a realization that happened within the past year or two. I don't remember its context — where I was, what I was doing, what specific matter was the occasion for the realization. I remember praying silently that some aspect of my work with Second Journey would contribute in some small way to the "coming of the Kingdom," the words we use in the Lord's Prayer. Then, as a postscript, I remember qualifying the sentiment: May I do this good thing. AND may I do it for the RIGHT REASONS. Not because I enjoy the work… which I did, immensely. Not because it taps my creativity… which it did, immensely. But because it will leave the world a better place.

Catholic theology, distinguishing between ethics and morality, holds that the merit of an action depends on the intention of the actor:

> So when you give to the needy, do not announce it with trumpets, as the hypocrites do in the synagogues and on the streets, to be honored by men. I tell you the truth, they have received their reward in full. But when you give to the needy, do not let your left hand know what your right hand is doing, so that your giving may be in secret. Then your Father, who sees what is done in secret, will reward you.[3]

When we act from a place deeper than ego, from the place of our deepest joy, we come into alignment with the divine spark in us and are absolved from asking further questions.

The Streaker

He lit out across the wide lawn,
naked, high stepping, arms flailing,
his pudgy trunk in constant search
for equilibrium. Sister

darted after him, his guardian angel
not seven years his senior, sailing
behind him, the sash of her white
linen shift floating in her wake.

Then catching up with him, she matched
his pace, letting him barrel on
giddily, in his riotous play,
just out of reach and rescue.

Then she turned him and steered him back.
And at the edge from which he'd launched,
scooped him up and — enfolding him —
whirled his giggling body round.

Who — knowing it would be such joy
to collapse into His cunning
Love — would not, like St. Francis — then
and there — strip and light out running?

— by Bolton Anthony

I was first introduced to *Awakening Osiris: The Egyptian Book of the Dead* through one of my spiritual teachers, who — during a retreat or gathering — would often read a passage from the book to help open our minds and our hearts to the profundity of the moment, much as one might use an inspirational poem. The author of this new translation and interpretation of the ancient Egyptian *Book of the Dead*, Normandi Ellis, suggests a more suitable title would be the "Book of Coming Forth by Day." Each chapter has a depth and power to it that puts our human existence into the vast context of the ebb and flow of all life forms throughout the ages, as we each come to understand who and what we really are. It's truly a remarkable book.

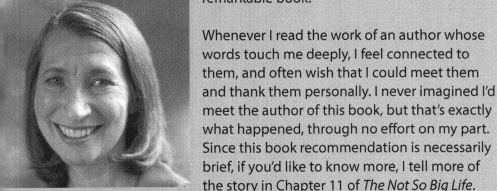

Sarah Susanka

Whenever I read the work of an author whose words touch me deeply, I feel connected to them, and often wish that I could meet them and thank them personally. I never imagined I'd meet the author of this book, but that's exactly what happened, through no effort on my part. Since this book recommendation is necessarily brief, if you'd like to know more, I tell more of the story in Chapter 11 of *The Not So Big Life*.

A thought leader, inspirational public speaker, and acclaimed architect, **Sarah Susanka** is the bestselling author of nine books, including *The Not So Big House*, *Home By Design*, and *The Not So Big Life: Making Room for What Really Matters*. Her books collectively weave together home and life design, revealing that a "Not So Big" attitude serves not only architectural aims, but life goals as well. Sarah received the 2007 Anne Morrow Lindbergh Award by the Lindbergh Foundation for outstanding individual achievement in making positive contributions to our world. She resides in Raleigh, North Carolina.

Making Room for Something New

by Sarah Susanka

Despite my early fascination with time's ability to morph and suspend a living moment as if it were a fly trapped in amber, I am also excruciatingly aware that all my life I've struggled with time — how to be in it effectively, how to engage it productively, and how to avoid being run over by it. For many years as a young adult, I was aware of my instant response when someone asked me how I was. "Too busy!" I'd say. Gradually it dawned on me that although I always thought the condition of *too-busyness* was temporary, it was in fact the most constant aspect of my world. And after a few more years of self-observation, I began to wonder if the condition was in fact my own creation. Was I somehow contriving my reality to be first and foremost too busy?

I noticed that although there were many things that had always inspired me and that I longed to do *when I had time* — such as writing a book, mastering another language, or learning to play the cello — these longings never got satisfied because I was ... too busy, too busy, too busy. So I started to wonder if perhaps there was some way I could make enough time to accomplish one of the items on my wish list. Since I'd wanted to be a writer before I knew much about anything else, I decided to build into my week some time to write. I decided to put it on the calendar, schedule it in, just like I would a meeting with

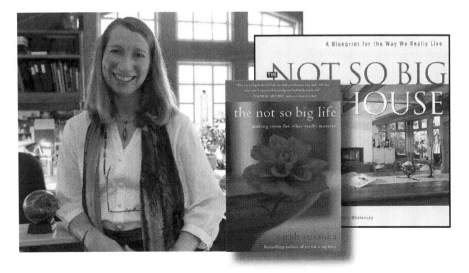

one of my clients, even though it seemed an outrageous act, given how busy I always was. I told myself I'd just have to live with the consequences; the one thing I wouldn't compromise was my writing time.

So began my Tuesday and Thursday morning meetings with myself and with my computer. Although I didn't realize it then, my life was about to change dramatically, and the keyboard would be a major player in that change. At first the purpose of these mornings was pretty fuzzy. I knew I wanted to write a book about architecture, my primary passion and career direction at the time, but I didn't know what form it would take. For several weeks I simply wrote to myself, in more or less a journal format, pondering the book's direction.

My father's early advice to me often echoed in my mind. He had wisely advised me, when I was a teenager and determined to become a fiction writer, that I should wait until I had something to say before becoming an author. During the past decade I'd frequently felt that I now had the appropriate level of expertise under my belt and was ready to say something, but paradoxically I believed that I no longer had the time to say it. My career was going full tilt, and I hardly had time to meet my architectural commitments let alone do anything else. It was only when I decided to question my belief in my own "too-busyness" that I discovered the time was there, ready and waiting. An Olivetti moment if ever there was one!

I simply needed to clarify for myself what part of my expertise I wanted to commit to paper. When I spoke in public about the designs of our homes — the focus of my architectural career — audiences seemed fascinated. What I described, in terms that made architecture accessible to everyone, was the power of good design to inspire us and affect our sense of well-being. I knew that there was much more significance to a house than merely the provision of shelter, and I wanted to impart what I knew about designing in all three dimensions — not just the floor plan, but the heights of spaces as well. Over my years of practice, I'd developed some language to help explain the various principles that architects use in their three-dimensional designs. It occurred to me that this might be the material I should write about.

I'd entered the field of architecture because I had always been profoundly affected by spatial experience — by the way beautifully designed buildings and spaces could transport me into a state of rapture, just as the Olivetti exhibition had. I had accumulated over my early life numerous memories of powerful spatial experiences that moved me deeply and that

Making Room for Something New

affected who I had become. And somehow, through describing my own passion for spatial experience, I'd been able to convey my enthusiasm to others.

After much deliberation, I decided to write down what I was already teaching in my public talks, describing in simple terms the principles I'd developed to help people of average means, who were not trained in design, to make their homes into more comfortable places to live, as well as truer expressions of themselves. As I started this process by making time for something I'd always longed to do, my world — all of it — started to shift in ways I could never have imagined.

The idea for the book led to my designing and building a new house for myself, to illustrate all the concepts I was writing about. I needed to show, in almost prototypical form, that it's possible to create a house for today by paring away the old, formal rooms, like the living room, dining room, and foyer, so that the dollars saved can be put into the spaces we REALLY use instead.

But what I wasn't expecting as I went about the design process was the amount of soul searching that went on as I tried to determine what spaces I personally desired. I'd designed hundreds of houses and additions for clients and knew that it was a pretty all-consuming process — almost like therapy, some people told me — but I thought it would be different for me because this was how I made my living. I already knew how to design a house. But I quickly found myself just as lost in the possibilities as any of my clients had been.

In my public presentations, I'd often bemoaned the fact that once we get married, all the space in the house is usually shared. If children arrive on the scene, they'll frequently be given their own rooms, yet parents, who often have very different tastes from each other, are forever joined at the hip when it comes to space for living. What would happen, I asked, if we allowed ourselves the luxury of a small amount of space that we could make completely personal, for nurturing that part of ourselves that longs to express itself, perhaps through a hobby or through contemplation — a place of one's own? I hadn't realized that for all those years I'd been speaking about a space that *I* longed for.

As the design evolved, I found myself daring to consider this possibility. I felt almost embarrassed, not quite sure if this was really OK. I wanted a place to meditate and to write in, but I didn't want it to be office-like at all. It was to be my sacred space, my place in which to start expressing my vibrant inner world. This was my first foray into bringing it out into the open and into built form, and the further along we got in the design process, the more certain I was that it was important and should be included.

I finally located this space at the very top of the house, in a sort of garret accessed by a ship's ladder, with a window low to the floor so that I could sit on my meditation cushion and look out across the expanse of the Mississippi Valley. As a lover of things geometrical, I'd designed the room to be a perfect equilateral triangle, so it had steeply sloping walls and was very cozy — a place not for standing and striding but for curling up with a good book or listening to a favorite piece of music.

The day I stepped into that space for the first time and sat down on my cushion to meditate, a most amazing thing happened. I felt as though the person sitting there — supposedly me — had been sitting there for eternity and would continue to sit there forever. There was a timeless, placeless connection to my true Self — the more aware and thus higher aspect of myself — and all the occasions I could recall of my being completely engaged in the moment were right there too. It was a profound experience indeed; and it had happened, in part at least, because I'd made a time and a place to be quiet and to listen to the wisdom of my own heart.

Over the next few months, with the Not So Big House prototype completed, the book of the same name started to take shape, and much of it was written in my attic space, my place of my own. What I discovered from the process of creating a place for my inner life is that when you make the time and the space for what you long to do, everything else shifts to accommodate it. In my experience it never works the other way around. If you wait until there's time to do what you want, you'll be waiting until your eighty-fifth birthday.

It never ceases to amaze me how insidious our conditioning is. I'm conditioned to be always too busy. For you it might be something else, something that seems equally real and equally frustrating. Just like the fish that doesn't realize it's surrounded by water because it's in it constantly, our conditioning is so much a part of our experience that we forget it's there, and we fall into the idea that the outer world is conspiring to keep us from doing what we want to do, when in fact our obstacles are self-generated.

Once you make the unequivocal internal commitment to do something — when you absolutely KNOW this is the time and the place to act — the world around you will shift in all sorts of apparently miraculous ways to make it happen. But they're not really miracles. This is the fluid nature of both life and consciousness. When your intentions are clear, events move to support them and to expand the ripple effect of your efforts.

Everything is always perfectly in balance when perceived from the perspective of the singular whole. And time, that elusive and enigmatic fourth dimension, isn't at all what we think it is. When we learn to engage it in a more conscious way, it can reveal an entirely new and vastly more amazing universe than we had realized is here, surrounding us in every moment of every day. We are, quite literally, fish in an ocean of time.[1]

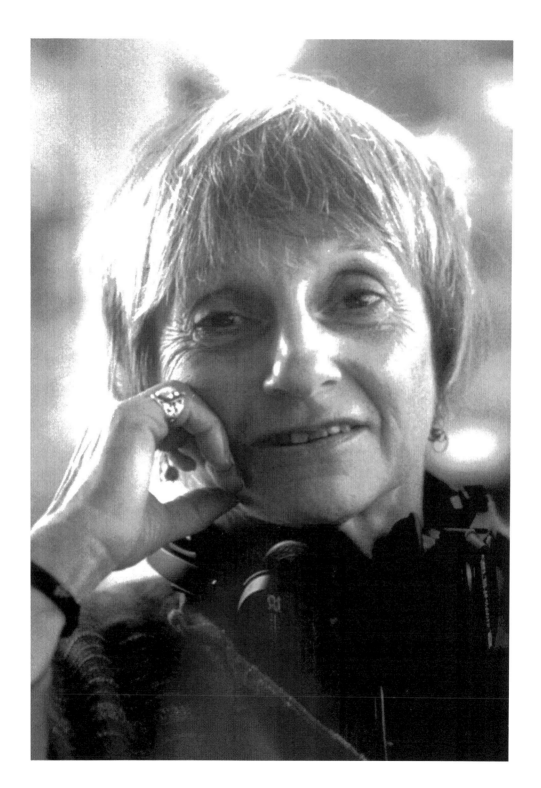

Honoring Our Elders

Connie Goldman: Mother Wisdom and the Aging Beat

I first met Connie Goldman when she was a reporter for National Public Radio, covering the "aging beat," as she described it. Actually, she had been the arts reporter before that, and her growing interest in artists and performers growing older had led her to a deepening interest in aging. At first she didn't get a lot of support for her "aging beat." But she persisted, and she has become a prominent journalistic voice, one of the most creative in our country, a national treasure, as the Japanese might put it.

When Connie first turned up in my office at the Brookdale Center on Aging in New York City, I immediately realized that I had found an ally: that is, someone who truly believed that later life could be a season of growth and positive change. I chuckle now when I think how young both she and I were at that time (30 years ago!). Yet, perhaps in proof of the "continuity theory of aging," I haven't changed my positive view and neither has she.

In the years since then, we're both older (I'm even on Medicare myself), but, as always, Connie is 15 years older than me and she remains a pioneer leading the path before me. But not only me. Connie is, and has been, a guide for all of us. In a professional group on aging and marketing in which we both participate (The Society), we have a nickname for Connie: "Mother Wisdom." The name could not be more apt.

Connie would certainly refuse any claim to wisdom, probably describing herself as a merely an interviewer, someone who asks questions and who listens carefully. That's all true. But it was also true for the very paradigm of wisdom, Socrates, who got in lots of trouble by asking questions.

Connie is not by nature a troublemaker but she is engaged in "disturbing the peace" because she asks deep, sometimes disturbing questions about aging. As she herself has advanced further into the territory of later life, her questions only get deeper — and sometimes more disturbing.

An earlier radio series she did was entitled "I'm Too Busy to Talk," and at that time she envisaged a side of positive aging which reflects activity, curiosity, and growth in new directions. All quite valid, and admirable. But there is more, and as she herself deepened the quest, she has become a one-woman testament to "conscious aging," which is something different from either "successful aging" (good health and social ties) or "productive aging" (contributing to the world around us). Connie's own aging has, without doubt, been "successful" and "productive." But that's not why I treasure her or why the interviews she has done have proved so influential. In recent years, Connie has probed the "hidden rewards of caregiving" (challenging the conventional thinking on this topic) and now she's exploring what it means to be one receiving care. In this deepening quest, she has paralleled with Ram Dass as he has done, moving from writing a book titled *How Can I Help?* to asking the (provocative) question: How can you help me? Ram Dass's question is not at all egocentric. Quite the opposite. It's an attempt to grapple with caregiving and the challenge of dependency. So it is with explorers like Ram Dass and Connie Goldman. They ask questions that challenge conventional thinking and make us reflect on our own path through later life.

The questions she asks, and the answers that she gets, have brought us all a deeper consciousness of what age can mean. In his *Letters to a Young Poet*, Rilke wrote, "Live the questions now. Perhaps you will then gradually without noticing it, live along some distant day into the answer." This is the trajectory of Mother Wisdom herself. The Psalmist tells us to "Number our days." My wish is that we should number, and treasure, the days of her life as Connie Goldman helps us all find a path with a heart.

— Harry R. Moody

It Will Come to Me

the word is there
i know it well
i will sound rusty chords
place my tongue just so
move my lips in aged patterns

the word is there
part of a thought
waiting for the word
to make it whole
it will do my bidding
in its own time

lost in the labyrinth
of a convoluted brain
it sits inert
in a cul-de-sac
a rock settled
deep in place
stubborn unyielding

it is not my first word
formed in an unmapped mind
it is one of many
saved from a lifetime
    listening
    sounding
    singing
the melody of language

the word sits poised to move
this word will tell you
what I need you to know

it is my word
i will speak it to you
wait with me until it comes
      — Dorthi Dunsmore[†]

[†] Published in *Celebrating Poets over 70*, M. Vespry and E. Ryan, editors (McMaster Centre for Gerontological Studies, 2010).

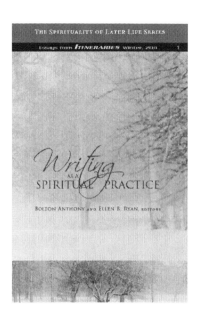

Writing as a Spiritual Practice

2011 Spring issue of Itineraries: *Selections and Supplements*

Plunging Inward for the Giving Words (NEW)
    by Ellen B. Ryan, Contributing Editor 77

The Tapestry of Your Life
    by Nora Zylstra-Savage 83

Writing in Groups
    by Paula Papky 87

Writing to Reclaim Identity in Dementia
    by Karen A. Bannister 93

Celebrating Poets Over 70
    by Marianne Vespry 101

Plunging Inward for the Giving Words

by Ellen B. Ryan

OLD AGE BRINGS CHANGE, more losses than gains, and an increasing awareness of death. Older adults can follow a path of growth in wisdom and compassion, or we can stagnate in isolation and despair.

One spiritual call in later life is to review our lives, seeking wisdom and a sense of wholeness. Another is to contribute to our world, especially to younger and future generations.

Writing can help us to clarify and meet these challenges. Writing is a spiritual practice through which we can contemplate, listen for quiet insights, be drawn to a sense of purpose, and engage in mindful service.

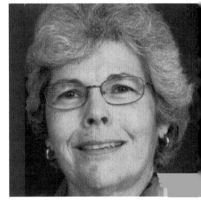

Current models of vital aging focus on healthy eating, physical exercise, mental exercise, adapting to losses, incorporating gains related to life experience, and engaging with life. The inner work of spirituality deepens our motivation to take on these responsibilities. Studies of centenarians highlight characteristics such as faith, hard work, family values, resilience, sidestepping adversity, and a sense of humor. We can develop motivation to live all the days of our lives by creating meaning at various life stages from active postretirement to frailty and finally to dying.

Journaling, writing for ourselves, can be central to spiritual practice in later life, a vehicle for reflection and prayer. In addition, some men and women may choose to write as part of their service to others. Here I will tell my own story to illustrate the importance of writing in later life, both for personal development and for contributing to society. The possibilities are endless, unique for each person responding to the invitation to write regularly.

Writing and Inner Work

It is looking at things for a long time that ripens you and gives you a deeper understanding.   — Vincent Van Gogh

You need only claim the events of your life to make yourself yours.
    — Florida Scott-Maxwell

I BEGAN KEEPING A JOURNAL while recovering from a car accident some years ago. Double vision and vertigo limited my ability to work and left me adrift. I could read for only brief periods, usually with enlarged font and text-to-speech computer adaptations. For pleasure reading I learned to listen to talking books. I felt especially cut off because I found myself physically uncomfortable in church for liturgy and could not do my accustomed spiritual reading.

My academic writing projects stalled. I was plagued by a recurring nightmare in which I searched madly for words while getting lost in a huge field of sunflowers. I could no longer spread papers out to consult while I wrote. Now I had to delegate reading and writing tasks to colleagues and students.

A friend introduced me to Julia Cameron's morning pages from *The Artist's Way* — write three pages each morning on any topic, just keep the pen moving. At first I wrote with big colored markers on every other line. Later my eyes allowed me to write more normally with a fine-tip marker in a spiral notebook. Soon writing and thinking with the journal became my way of organizing each day as well as contemplating my life.

At first the pages filled with all sorts of complaints. Gradually, some perspective emerged. I began to write about how my situation could be worse, about all the supports I enjoyed, and the potential for learning valuable lessons through these experiences. Unable to pray much at the time, I began to listen during my writing sessions for spiritual insights — and the more I listened the calmer and more trusting I became. My enforced solitude and quiet non-reading life became a gift of time for my journal — paying more and more attention to the moment, nature, myself, and other people.

After a while I could read a couple of pages a day. These were selected from books increasingly well-chosen for their readable fonts and stimulus for contemplation. I scribbled away, reflecting on the few printed words I had managed to absorb and their applications to my current life, to my life as part of humanity, to all life on earth. I learned later that reading in small doses followed by reflection has a long spiritual tradition — "lectio divina." Through this process, I faced my feelings, counted my blessings daily, and asked myself more and more fundamental questions. As Doris Gumbach wrote in her late-life memoir, "Keeping a journal thins my skin. I feel open to everything, aware, charged by the acquisition of intensity."

Since then, journaling about other spiritual practices after each episode — prayer, liturgy, long walks, physical exercise, church groups, meditation, volunteer work — has deepened and supported these disciplines over the long term.

Life review is central to personal growth in later life. Writing regularly about the highs and lows of our lives — past, present, and possible futures — can lead us through the inner work needed to claim that life, that evolving self. Looking at ourselves in this manner gives us a foundation for reaching out to others. As I continued to dig for memory treasure in my life story, I became more aware of the Author of life.

Through Julia Cameron's *The Artist's Way* and Natalie Goldberg's *Writing Down the Bones*, I discovered that writing exercises would take me repeatedly into life review. Stirring my imagination and heart, these starters move my pen ahead of my thinking mind. I started to incorporate sensory details, metaphor, and word play. Kathleen Adams' *Journal to the Self* offered enticing suggestions about making lists (e.g., where I would like to travel, my favorite celebrations), writing letters (to be sent or not), and composing dialogues between myself and another (e.g., mentor/parent, God, nature, a specific author or an inanimate object).

After months of journaling and using writing exercises, a half-waking dream made clear to me that I should learn to write poetry. During the dream I realized how well poetry would fit with my ongoing reading and writing impairments — just a few words, with plenty of white space. I awoke from the dream calmly confident that I would be able to say what I needed to say through this unfamiliar medium.

Not knowing how to proceed, I wrote about the dream in my journal, and realized it would be wise to take a course. Ironically, the course I chose did not involve the anticipated lectures. Participants were expected to bring 15 copies of their poem to a workshop for critiques by group

The Road Now

Retiring from paid work
I stop to see where I am

follow the echoes
of projects heralded
for grit and wit

touch the ribbed weave
of disciplines colourful
in their crossing

sniff the ricochet
of novel thoughts
tearing through
tough peels
of assumptions

taste the chocolate cherry joy
of collaborations where
three minds surpass
possibility

What road now
worth the pilgrimage

— Ellen B. Ryan

members and by the leader/poet. Instead of learning about iambic pentameter and poetry of the ages, I was soon writing for the group's gentle critique. My entry into creative expression with the mutual support of a writing group was exhilarating.

My experience of writing poetry has been spiritual. I write in my journal, participate in a writing group, use writing exercises, pay close attention to nature and people, make lists of images and startling words, and listen for the muse. Creating a small database of colorful verbs (e.g., juxtapose, catapult, scrounge, trumpet) has been a special delight. Yet, when a poem begins to emerge, it comes as a gift of words from God. For me, creativity is both listening prayer and expressive prayer. Once I have the initial skeleton of a poem, I am learning strategies to craft ever better final versions. Stretching myself in this new creativity is nourishing. Some of my poems appear in this book.

Writing is an act of discovery. The regular discipline of journaling stretches the spirit and opens my mind, reduces my fears to mere words, and highlights my blessings. Through journaling, I return repeatedly to basic questions of identity and to basic values, especially awe, gratitude, and love.

I wanted to choose words that even you would have to be changed by. — Adrienne Rich

Words lead to deeds ... They prepare the soul, make it ready, and move it to tenderness. — St. Teresa of Avila

Writing As Service

WRITING CAN BECOME A CALLING, central to how we choose to age with spirit. Journaling usually combines inner reflection with decisions for action — in the domain of writing and beyond.

Once the inner work progresses, we may wish to express our social voices. This can start with more thoughtful letters to family and friends, may extend to letters to the editor or newsletter/Web site contributions. Personal writing can progress into memoir, history, essay, poetry, and fiction to share with friends and relatives or to publish in magazines, Web sites, and books.

When I took early retirement, I deliberated at length in the journal about my postretirement calling. Over time, I developed the goal to learn new kinds of writing. I had already begun to address storytelling and storywriting of elders in my academic research, partly because I could no longer focus on my usual complex analyses. Partly, however, this was a natural late-career shift from the theory underlying problematic communication with frail elders to application: how to facilitate mutually rewarding communication.

Eventually, I identified my passion for these years: "writing to learn, teach, and inspire others." I am committed to improving my poetic skills and to submitting poems regularly, if sparingly, for publication. I edit the Writing Down Our Years series of inexpensive publications highlighting the writing of older adults, especially memoirs, grandparent–grandchild stories, caregiving stories, and poetry. I offer writing workshops and initiate writing groups.

With colleagues and students, I continue to explore creative ways to elicit and write down the stories and poems of elders who are physically and/or cognitively frail. My writing for professionals fosters enthusiasm for hearing, reading, and eliciting such stories. Finally, I host a Web site on Writing, Aging and Spirit for a broad audience of older adults and aging professionals to foster hope and connections through story.

When we write as service, we can be entertainer, chronicler, historian, social commentator, educator, advocate, and/or activist.

In conclusion, writing is working as a spiritual practice when it enriches our sense of self in community and invigorates our service to others.

Like life, aging is a choice, a series of choices. On reaching 70, the acclaimed spiritual writer and social activist Joan Chittister reflects on these choices in *The Gift of Years: Growing Old Gracefully*. Brief, engaging essays address expected topics such as meaning, adjustment, relationships, letting go, memories, forgiveness, and wisdom. Importantly, she also examines topics less often linked to old age, such as accomplishment, possibility, dreams, agelessness, and the future.

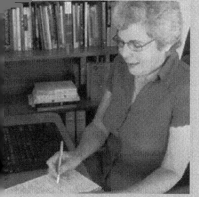

Ellen B. Ryan

What I like best about this book is how Chittister outlines the choices so clearly — each essay concludes with a statement of "the burden of these years" and "the blessing of these years." The gift of these years is the invitation to become fully alive, to grow deeply, and to finally know what really matters. If we don't give in to our limitations, we can reach out to others in ways the world so desperately needs. This final affirmation — that the world awaits the legacy of those burnished by old age — strikes me as her most significant message. We need to grow spiritually in old age, not only for ourselves but for the sake of the world.

Ellen B. Ryan is Professor Emeritus at McMaster University in Hamilton, Ontario. In addition to numerous journal articles on communication, aging, and health, her publications include the Writing Down Our Years Series (1998–2010) and Ability Speaks: Talking with a Person with Disability (2009). She hosts the Web site and blog on Writing, Aging and Spirit (see www.writingdownouryears.ca).

The Tapestry of Your Life

by Nora Zylstra-Savage

PERSONAL STORIES HAVE THE POWER to entertain, heal, and connect you with your own personal truths and beliefs. Reflecting, recording, and sharing stories is an exercise in discovery and validation that is vital for your own and others' spiritual and emotional well-being. Life stories are the best connection to the past and are important to share with each other, family, and especially the younger generation. They're a window into a different time period.

Before you decide which type or style of memoir is best suited to your life experiences and your writing style, it is extremely helpful to identify the major events in your life. Stop for a moment now to "prime the pump" with the following exercise which I call "Creating a Life Circle."

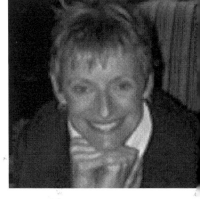

Start with a large sheet of blank paper and draw a large circle to the outer edge of the page. Draw a ½" rim on the inside of this circle. Next divide the circle into eight equal Parts. Take your current age and divide it by eight — this number (the years number) will be the number of years represented in each Part. Start with your birth year and add the years number. So if you were born in 1931 and your years number is 10, the first Part's heading would be 1931–1941; each subsequent heading would be 10 years more until the current year. This allows you to jot down all the major events in your life within the correct Part and to observe at a glance the events of your life. If there are blank areas, knowing what came before and after can help you figure out what is missing. If you are planning to only write about a particular time period or a specific set of experiences, such as having survived cancer, that span of time can be extrapolated and expanded into a new circle and further divided into smaller time periods for more detail.

Once your life circle has been filled out, you are ready to decide what type of memoir best suits your actual experiences. You may choose from the highlights of your life, an autobiography, a partial memoir, or a thematic or a reflective one.

> Stacked and scattered,
> tall and tumbling,
> mounds of records,
> each a thought, a feeling,
> or a melody.
> — Sigrid Kellenter[1]

The highlights of your life, or a life review, encourages you to write about your strongest memories which normally represent a few stories from each life stage or milestone. This form is the most diverse of memoir types, as it allows for a variety of formats and styles in one book. It can be a collection of events, relationship stories, family traditions, moments in time, character sketches, social and political essays, poems, recipes, photos, sketches, or memorabilia; and it normally is presented in chronological order, by theme, or a combination of both. If you can't remember all the details of a certain event or have gaps between years, or if you simply prefer a variety of writing styles and memoir inclusions, the "highlights" memoir might be your best option.

The second type of memoir is the autobiography, which normally spans from birth to the present day. The autobiography is a detailed factual account of your whole life, which usually adheres to one style of writing. Each chapter could represent a year or several years; chronological order is usually maintained. Photos or poems are not usually included in an autobiography; however, many have a photo collection Part, either in the middle or the end of the book.

> Tapping the trees of memories
> boiling down the sap
> of long and challenging years.
> — Helen Vanier[2]

A partial memoir represents a specific period of time in your life. Many areas and periods of time could be chosen. Consider writing only about your childhood. *Liar, Liar, Your Pants on Fire* is one good example; here the author, Mary Cook, writes about her childhood years growing up in the country during the depression. If you were a teacher, you may only want to write about all your teaching years, including your training, the different schools and grades you've taught, and the many personal challenges, highlights, and insights that you've experienced. Consider writing about living in a particular community, town, or city. What about your struggles and triumphs with a sickness or disease? Another partial memoir could detail your experiences during war time, which could include your decision to enlist, the many reactions to this, your training, deployment, and return. Your war stories could also include current reflections on your past experiences or the topic of war. A partial memoir allows you to focus and delve deeper into particular topics, experiences, or periods of time.

Thematic memoirs are another style that you may choose. There are several types within this category. Thematic memoir topics — music, family traditions, travel, clothes, appliances, friends, cars (the list is endless) — continue to repeat themselves throughout your life. All the stories selected must hook onto the theme chosen. An example might be: my life told through the clothes I wore. A book with this theme — *Love, Loss, and What I Wore* — was written and illustrated by Ilene Beckerman. Other thematic titles might include: all the cars I've ever owned, or my spiritual journey.

Internal life challenges are also a choice in this thematic memoir style. You may choose to write more than one thematic life story. Themes could include addictions, betrayal, responsibility, disabilities, familial struggles, life lessons — this list, too, goes on and on. For this type, you need to identify your theme and then consider stories that represent your journey or evolution. These memoirs tend to be the most powerful, as they normally represent universal struggles that resonate with everyone's life in one way or another. An excellent book that provides the structure for you to identify personal themes is *Writing the Memoir* by Judith Barrington.

The final type of memoir is reflective. There are two different styles. For those of you who enjoy philosophizing about life, here is an opportunity to share insights about your life or life in general through metaphoric poetry or prose. You might compare your life to a river with its many branches, depths, speeds, directions, and obstacles. Or you may be fascinated with plants, the environment, the elements, the weather, nature, or even nonliving elements. Imagine your life as a sports car, an orchestra, a color, or even a boat. The other way of approaching a reflective memoir is to identify all the major turning points or milestones in your life. Write about each event followed by a reflection describing your feelings, decisions, insights, and directions based on the event.

> The driveway is haunted by bodies
> of cars that rust in weeds and rubble
> on the edges of towns where nobody goes.
> — Robert Currie[3]

There are many story styles available for you to choose from. The best thing you can do for yourself, your family, or your friends and even the community is to START. Family members have died, and often with them die irreplaceable stories. A vital part of our social, cultural, and family history will be forgotten and lost. Life stories help you understand your past, acknowledge the present, and create new possibilities for your future. The time is now — Put it in writing!

Iowa

What a strange happiness.
Sixty poets have gone off drunken, weeping
    into the hills,
I among them.
There is no one of us who is not a fool.
What is to be found there?
What is the point in this?
Someone scrawls six lines and says them.
What a strange happiness.
    — Robert Sward[†]

[†] Published in *Celebrating Poets over 70*, M. Vespry and E. Ryan, editors (McMaster Centre for Gerontological Studies, 2010).

Writing in Groups

by Paula Papky

For me, writing in a group has always been about discovery: who I am, where I fit in the world, what to go on with, and what to leave behind. I want to discover what guides I have in this stage of life, old age.

I have been writing with a group of women, every other Thursday, since 2001. An amazing community has come into being through our writing together, one of deep trust and consolation and support but also one of creativity and risk-taking and confidence. We have experienced together times of sorrow for loss and many moments of hilarity. All of this has come about because, when we get together, we practice fast writing for a set period of time, followed by reading aloud by those who choose to do so. There's nothing like unedited writing, thoughts hot off the page, to inspire a sense of gratitude, and sometimes awe.

Any Writing Can Be Fast Writing

The idea of writing in a group occurred to me nearly 20 years ago when I read Natalie Goldberg's *Writing Down the Bones*.[1] I was captivated by the process of fast writing that she described. Remembering one's life story was a big part of fast writing. Soon I was using it for the many writing projects that my work in pastoral ministry required, particularly sermon preparation and the creation of liturgy and prayers for Sunday services as well as homilies for funerals and weddings. I used it for writing newspaper articles and newsletters in the church and in the wider community, and for drafts of essays in courses I took. I found myself keeping a journal and writing poetry and even turning to fiction writing. There was something unfathomable, bottomless, about the process. It helped me make the critical decision to leave pastoral ministry for a time, and eventually, to return to teaching high school English, where, of course, I gave my students daily opportunities for self-discovery through fast writing. The key to such writing was always having good springboards, of which Natalie Goldberg supplied many in *Writing Down the Bones* and her subsequent books.

None of this was writing in groups, though. That came about when a friend, who knew I was writing, recommended *Journal to the Self* by Kathleen Adams.[2] It contained more springboards and intriguing exercises for self-discovery. I was so excited by the two practices, fast writing and keeping a journal, that I wanted to teach their use to others. I offered a Saturday morning course, titled "Writing for Spiritual Discovery," in a church I had joined. Only women turned up — 12 women, aged from mid-thirties to late seventies.

Writing Builds Community

THE PROCESS WE FOLLOWED was fast writing followed by immediate reading aloud. For 12 weeks we built trust, increased confidence, laughed and cried, and put into words our deepest thoughts, our prayers, our lyric poems. These weeks were so engaging that when we finished the course, half of us wanted to do it again. And we did, for years, on Saturday mornings. Muffins and coffee, the quiet scratching of pens on the page, the reading — we learned a lot about ourselves and each other and our relationship with the Divine. Women who had, as they described, written only grocery lists and dates on calendars, were writing poems as well as journal entries. The fear of having nothing to say disappeared, and a small community took shape. That's what writing in groups does: It builds community. It helps discover community where before there was mere acquaintance among people. Age barriers disappear. The shy discover a voice. The extrovert learns to listen. The nonwriters become committed writers/explorers.

Now, 15 years later, I have practiced writing in groups with teachers, poets, high school students, fiction writers, and for a few weeks, the elderly (some with dementia) living in a care residence. Most recently I have used fast writing in Bible Study groups, as ways of entering into a story from Scripture, almost as if we are writing ourselves into the narratives.

In the Bible Study, we use fast writing to have a dialogue with Jesus or Zacchaeus or the Syro-Phoenician woman. Or we take the voice of a bystander in the crowd and retell the story. These group writing practices have engaged both men and women. Certainly they have drawn our church community closer together. The commitment to confidentiality frees us up to enter deep waters, to take risks and to express feelings — an experience some of the men found unnerving but always enlightening.

Starting a Fast-Writing Group

THE GROUP I WRITE WITH NOW most often is a dozen women aged 50-something to nearly 100. It began with a few members of a book club that read together Ellen Jaffe's book, *Writing Your Way: Creating A Personal Journal*.[3] When they decided they wanted to try some of her ideas, they invited her to lead them through a session. Little did she or they know that their writing in a group would become a way of life. A couple of members invited me to come along because they knew I had experience in writing with a group and fast writing. And here we all are, a decade later. We spend two hours fast writing and reading aloud. We share the leadership in an informal way, taking turns bringing a springboard poem or suggesting a topic. Recent topics from these sessions have been: homesickness; mountains; what I carry with me; arrivals and departures; the color green; my outdoor childhood. Nothing is too trivial. What one person writes and reads aloud may spark a memory or an image for someone else to explore in the next 10-minute plunge into the page.

We have found out a great deal about ourselves, our community of 12, our creativity, and our wisdom. Over and over we have experienced wonder, which some would call the sacred and others a sense of belonging to something larger. Our discovery has often led to discussion that is deeply spiritual and honors our various faith traditions — Christian, Jewish, as well as those with no particular religious affiliation but with a keen sense of the presence of the sacred in the moments of our lives.

There are a few important guidelines for a writing group like ours to begin and flourish, but only a few. After that, the discoveries are endless.

Most important is to build trust. Some of us knew each other in the group from the start, while others were strangers. We left nothing to chance where building trust was concerned. At our first session we promised each other confidentiality. Nothing that anyone wrote and read aloud was to be repeated outside the group. If you are starting this kind of writing group, it can take time to go around the circle and have each one, in turn, commit to this promise, but do it anyway, even if you are all friends to begin with. And remind each other regularly about that debt to confidentiality. One way to raise the issue occasionally is for people to express thanks for that gift, for the freedom to be honest or to explore a difficult issue without worrying about their story being told by someone else. My experience with this initial covenant is that trust develops quickly and deeply. Each member is able to discover and express a full range of feelings in a confidential setting.

Well, by now you may be wondering if this writing in a group is actually psychoanalysis. It is not. That's a second boundary we put in place as the group formed. When someone reads aloud a piece of fast writing, or talks about what they were writing, our response is to say, "Thank you." We don't try to correct or fix anyone. No one says, "Well you should just…" or "Why don't you…" We just say, "Thank you." I think gratitude is one of the great gifts of our writing together. No one has to shape up or settle down or all those parental-sounding responses to self-discovery. The writing is what it is. And we're grateful for it.

And what, exactly, is it, this writing we do in a group? It's fast and unedited, stream-of-consciousness writing. We have Natalie Goldberg to thank for this process. Don't cross out or correct spelling or steer your thoughts, she tells us. Feel free to produce the worst writing in the universe! It's just writing practice, isn't it? So, she advises, practice making your hand move across the page, right across the margins, if you like. Set a timer for 10 minutes and write like crazy. When the time is up, stop. Then read aloud if you want to. Then go for another 10 minutes, and another 10.

Begin with Remembering

WE FIND, EVEN NOW, there's no better place to begin than Natalie Goldberg's, "I remember." Whenever your pen stops, just repeat "I remember" and keep going. Remember as much as you can: the sights, sounds, scents, tastes, and touches of your life. Be specific. Name the cities, streets, beaches, stores. And sometimes, when your pen stops, try "I don't remember" and keep going. It can be like turning over a rock and discovering what was hidden or half-buried.

Recently we began by making a list of a dozen "seasons of my life" and chose one to follow up in fast writing that began, "I remember." Lists are great prompters of memories. Remember skipping through recess in grade five, playing marbles in the spring, playing softball in the field, skating on the pond, building forts? And lately, we have discovered that taking a particular year and a season of childhood or adolescence yields lots of memories. As we age, we cherish these memories and can be guided by them to be more playful, more open to new experiences. And we can consider our lives' turning points and how they changed us.

It is in Kathleen Adams' book *Journal to the Self* that these starting places for writing are called "springboards." She provides dozens of places to begin in using writing for personal growth, including lists, dialogues, and stepping stones. Her exercises aren't intended for fast writing particularly, but that's how we worked through them, and it was very rich.

After all these years of writing together, our group's favorite springboards come from lyric poems. Someone in the group brings a poem by a published poet and reads it aloud (sometimes more than once, sometimes more than one reader) and we each grab a line we like and run with it. The line may get repeated several times as a way to keep the writing going and to give it a lovely unity and coherence. Many a piece of fast writing has turned into a poem through the repeated line or image from someone else's poem: Lucille Clifton's "I am running into a new year"[4] and Mary Oliver's "The Summer Day,"[5] for instance, we have used several times.

Companionship for Self-Discovery

SOMETIMES IN A PIECE OF FAST WRITING, a member of the group gets into deep water, into hidden depths they didn't set out to explore. This is where writing in a group is so liberating. If we find ourselves writing and reading aloud about loss, others are listening, withholding judgment. The writing group is a listening ear, with the possibility for consolation and compassion. If someone discovers in writing a new path to take, the possibility for healing, the writing group rejoices. These responses help to build self-esteem. In our group, we are learning how not to apologize before we read aloud, how not to preface our reading with a disclaimer like, "This isn't very good" or "I have no idea where this is going." We keep an informal list of some of our earlier disclaimers. We joke that we're going to number them and put the list on a T-shirt someday, so we only have to point to one of them before reading. We can grieve in this group. We can laugh. We don't need to apologize.

As we age, what more can be discovered about oneself by writing in a group than by writing alone? It may be that we push ourselves a little harder when others in our group are encouraging us. That woman who came to my first writing workshop, having written only cards and notes on calendars, is still writing poems. She is in her 99th year, nearly blind, and living in a retirement home, but she's still writing poems. Because of her limited vision, she has to wait until someone comes into her room who can write the poems down, but she's still writing. For all of us in this writing group, she has been an important mentor. Her poems about aging reveal her authentic voice, her unflinching gaze at her past and present. She's not afraid to write about loss, aging, sex, sisterhood, moving house,

God and her faith. She inspires and encourages our group, even now that she lives an hour away and can no longer write with us. And she continues to inspire the many others who have read the poems she has published, including her self-published book, *Light All Around Me* (edited by Ellen B. Ryan, whose article appears elsewhere in this anthology).

There is a deep well of wisdom available to those who gather in a group to write. We all want to know, especially as we age, what really matters in life — what to carry forward and what to leave behind. And here, month after month, year after year, we hear from a dozen writers, our trusted friends, what makes life precious and how each one has discovered those treasures of the heart.

In our group, some are retired teachers, a couple are counselors, some are published writers, and all are voracious readers and love words. We trust one another's wisdom, distilled from years of reading widely and from our lives' experiences. Our writing sessions, between 10-minute writing practices, include conversations about ideas. Of course, given our ages (fifties to nineties) we are learning about aging but also, because it pops up in our writing, about childhood and play and creativity and a hundred other subjects. *Always*, through our poem springboards, we are in touch with that wider community of writers, treating Emily Dickinson, May Sarton, Mary Oliver, and many other poets, male and female, as our mentors and guides in life.

Sometimes, writing in a group, we experience that relatively rare feeling of awe. Perhaps it comes as goose bumps when one of our oldest members writes about aging with devastating honesty. It may happen when someone writes and shares what an experience in the world of nature was like, what a particular place was like. Some in our group would describe these moments of rare insight as experiences of the sacred, of meeting the Holy One, of being touched by God. Others would shy away from God-language and might describe feeling very small in the face of something large and mysterious.

Because all of us in the group are exploring our lives and what meaning they have, these moments happen more often than in daily life. Our responses in such breakthrough moments are common responses to awe: tenderness, sympathy, gratitude. We encourage each other, console each other, hope for each other, trust each other. We are patient with slow growth, compassionate with setbacks, eager for news of the inner life. We cheer each other on for the apt word here, the resonant image there, and the courage to move that hand across the page without stopping.

Writing to Reclaim Identity in Dementia

by Karen A. Bannister

"Who will I be when I die?" – Christine Bryden

HE GREETS ME AT THE DOOR with a shy smile and a gracious, if anxious, hello. Still in his pajamas, he searches my face and I am immediately aware of his confusion. Declines in short-term memory mean he approaches me unprepared for my visit and uncertain of just who I am. He has Alzheimer's disease. An impeccable storyteller, we get together once a week to complete, for his wife, a collection of his exciting stories — as a young war refugee in Europe, as a young man coming to Canada, as a successful gerontologist and an award-winning skier. His speech, which I tape record and then later type into prose, is animated and often filled with great pride.

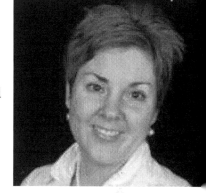

Alzheimer's has for him, as for so many others, caused problems with memory, language, and other abilities. It has become difficult to find the right words in conversation, to anticipate aspects of the day, and to avoid confusion when subjected to out-of-the-usual experiences like busy public spaces, large crowds, and phone calls from telephone solicitors. Many individuals with Alzheimer's, or related forms of dementia, retreat from social interaction to avoid confronting newly patronizing expectations and revealing their impairments to themselves and others. Fewer meaningful social interactions can have a profound effect on the evolution of an individual's sense of self.

> *"It is as if knowledge of the disease immediately cloaks me in invisibility."*[1]

This article examines the social position of individuals with dementia and suggests writing as a means to affirm selfhood. By using quotations from our study of the memoirs written by nine individuals living and growing with dementia, my colleagues and I advocate for listening to such voices when constructing approaches to caregiving.

The Social Position of Individuals with Dementia

DEMENTIA IS A DARK BEAST; it means the progressive deterioration of cognitive functioning due to Alzheimer's and related diseases. Impairments, usually beginning in the memory center, can move across areas of the brain responsible for language, vision, movement, and judgment. Loved ones may see the individual transformed as these impairments manifest themselves in recent memory loss, periods of mental confusion, reduced ability to assess risk, hallucinations, depression, and insomnia. The sufferer must confront this difficult time, to learn to cope with changing abilities and a reduced role in social conversation. Oral communication can be difficult: Word-finding and memory difficulties impair fluent speech and decrease an individual's confidence in conversation. Impaired vision, judgment, and emotional disturbance similarly restrict one's authority in social interactions.

> *I wrote to clarify for myself what was going on with me and in me.*[2]

Stereotypes are, in many ways, what guide our interactions with others. We come to a conversation with a set of expectations dependent on preconceived ideas. The dementia sufferer may be expected to be incompetent, no longer "present" and somehow childlike or in need of the continual intervention of others. Negative stereotypes can lead people to become apprehensive and unsure in the presence of different or "diseased" people and to alter their style of communication.

> Another really crazy thing about Alzheimer's, nobody really wants to talk to you any longer. They're maybe afraid of us.[3]

> Some friends and family seem to fear coming close to us to touch our true spirits. Perhaps they are uncomfortable, because they know instinctively that we are now different and they believe that their relationship with us has changed.[4]

> I have become keenly aware of a patterned response from some individuals as soon as they find out I have Alzheimer's disease. They switch their eye contact and attention to whomever I am with.[5]

These perceptions can create poor social interactions.

> Isolation is a real problem for us. Many of us feel that some people even think dementia is contagious! We don't see many friends any more. It seems as if people treat us differently now, because they know we have dementia, and they don't know what to do. Maybe they are worried about us saying something odd or doing something bizarre? Often we feel like we are being watched in case we do the wrong thing.[6]

Without constructive interactions, the person with dementia becomes stalled in the process of expressing a social identity, in counteracting the negative expectations of others, and in working through the meanings of the dementia experience. For example, losses of social and familial roles require emotional resolution and understanding. People usually rely on positive dialogue with close others to find this kind of resolution or meaning.

Writing and Dementia

PEOPLE WHO WRITE about their experiences find in this process an opportunity to engage with others and to explore meaning. This therapeutic process can facilitate the integration of diagnosis and altered abilities into a new sense of self. Through writing in a journal or for others, an individual can achieve clarity, empowerment, and new roles. By transforming emotion and images into words, a person can reorganize the way a traumatic event is remembered, contemplated, and even forgotten. Humor, a valuable device, can enable new perspectives through the creative use of language and analogy (e.g., "When I hurt, I yell, which is what I've been doing for several years now, and it's food for thought, at least, an Alzheimer's picnic").[7]

> I am working today, tapping at this keyboard with little time left, in an attempt to understand who I was and what is left.[8]

The act of writing, often faring better than speech, can foster remembering, mirror the ups and downs of life with the disease, and teach coping skills.

> The words in my brain are silent, and the flood of sentences begins only when my pen unleashes a flood of writing memory.[9]

> Watching my spelling, especially when it goes out of control, is a way I keep tabs on Ol' Alzheimer's.... I use it as a fingerprint of what is happening in my brain.[10]

> In the other, slower world where I write on paper or directly on the computer, vocabulary is more fluid and I often surprise myself when the perfect word finds its way into the sentence without effort.[11]

Individuals with illness or disability have a unique need to find expression in writing; they may feel that their voice has been taken from them by a medical diagnosis and the expectations of others. Writing can be a means to reclaim voice, to put a face on a disease, to connect with others living with the same condition, to educate others, and to advocate for social change. By constructing illness narratives, individuals can actively remake an identity.

Writing Through Metaphor to Elaborate Insights

CREATIVE LANGUAGE USE CAN HELP people with dementia better understand their feelings. The metaphor is used to create the image for the reader, but in deconstructing the image into words, the writer benefits from greater clarity. These dementia narratives demonstrate ample use of metaphor.

> In the swings of my emotion, from sunlight into ever blackening moonlight…[12]

> The interiors and exteriors of the world flash before me but I cannot find ways to open them.[13]

> The disease works slowly, destroying the mind, stealing life in a tedious silent dance of death.[14]

> I feel as if I am sitting in my grandmother's living room, looking at the world through her lace curtains. From time to time, a gentle wind blows the curtains and changes the patterns through which I see the world.[15]

Reflecting on complex thoughts and ideas with the help of the written word creates insight. The dementia writers seem to arrive at a new sense of awareness and personhood.

My friend, the impeccable storyteller, gained much from our sessions, especially a sense of comfort in reliving the memories of what makes him a successful, vital, and unique human being. Suddenly diagnosis had context, and the context was his vibrant life.

> As I read over this book…I realize how far I have come psychologically, if not intellectually. *Living in the Labyrinth* was written in a state of grief such as I'd never experienced, and it jumps out at me as I read back over the pages.[16]

> I have a life that can be either frustrating and frightening, or peaceful and submissive. The choice is mine. I choose to take things moment by moment, thankful for everything that I have, instead of raging wildly at the things that I have lost.[17]

> It is now 2004, and I am still here, and it has been quite a journey of understanding, of seeing more clearly who I am now, who I am becoming, and who I will be when I die.[18]

Writing Provides Empowerment

THROUGH THE ACT OF WRITING, an individual, sharing his identity, becomes "writer," "storyteller," and "teacher." These new roles provide feelings of accomplishment and purpose that are empowering and can elevate self-esteem.

My friend was able to embody valued roles — teacher, mentor, and storyteller. I believe he was able to re-establish himself as a competent social partner and a contributing member of society. Our interactions reminded him of his many accomplishments and also his likes, dislikes, beliefs, motivations, and inner feelings. This process can serve to reaffirm the existing personality, which may have been lost in feelings of lowered self-worth.

Empowerment is also derived from the control that writing provides. An individual, able to control the words on the page and to direct oneself (and often a caregiver) in an activity, finds an opportunity for enhancing self-esteem.

Working on a Story Project

A STORY PROJECT IS AN OPPORTUNITY to record family history, but also an exercise in affirming an individual's identity. You may begin by encouraging your loved one to record thoughts and ideas in a personal journal, either in written or oral form (as in recording thoughts with a tape recorder). By introducing the story project in this way, you encourage the incorporation of personal reflection and thoughts in the recall of stories. Individuals with dementia work best in well-lit, uncluttered, and quiet environments. Technology can provide great assistance as handwriting declines. Many of the writers cited here made use of tape recorders and computers.

An encouraging environment is important. It is useful to tell family and friends about the writer's story project and encourage them to participate by sparking story ideas or sharing their own memories. Story ideas can come from a number of sources: engaging in pleasurable activities, creating a memory book or box of treasured items, or just talking. To spark ideas, use active listening techniques with open posture, sit close and maintain eye contact, ask questions and paraphrase important information, make use of open-ended questions, read sections of writing back and ask the individual to fill in the blanks or expand. It is especially important to provide the person with the opportunity to direct the conversation and the duration of the activity. This includes understanding that some days and hours in the day are better than others; let individuals set their own limits. Regardless of the extent of support provided, the facilitator's goal is to empower the person with dementia to tell his or her own story in his or her own words and for these words to be recorded.

Conclusion

WRITING ENABLES THE INDIVIDUAL living with dementia to engage in positive social interaction with others, which enhances social identity. Writing can be done at any time and in any time frame. It hides one's disability and enables thoughts to become fully expressed without interruption and the fear of immediate rejection.

The writers we have quoted in this article are exemplary human beings who have written powerful reflections of their experiences. They have successfully come to resolve issues of social identity and taken on new and important roles. These individuals are growing positively with dementia; they are achieving new insight and awareness and passing this wisdom on to others. They have joined a community of readers and other writers and in so doing are breaking down stereotypes of "dementia sufferer."

While most people will not publish their work, writing is an activity that can be accomplished by all. The level of outside assistance required may differ for each person. Some people with dementia may need to have others write their words for them and reconstruct ideas to achieve clarity. An especially attractive aspect of writing is that it hides this process, ensuring that the final product is a complete thought ready for consumption, even for the most ill. While the authors cited here were in an early to moderate stage of dementia, facilitated life storytelling/writing and group poetry writing in long-term care facilities suggests that individuals in late-stage dementia can also participate in facilitated writing exercises.

Missing

He stands before me every day and
I can't tell who is here
I miss
who is absent

Here's nothing of the lusty
red hot fury of concentration
steam and sweat of heavy work

No rush to do
only impatience

with an unfamiliar voice,
accent
question
printed sheet
painted symbol All seem threats
him
What hums in his chest?
What presses on his frowning brows?
What word grasps the wish
but comes out twisted?
What name lost and
lost again
has disappeared?
                      — Phyllis Hotch[†]

[†] Published in *Celebrating Poets over 70*, M. Vespry and E. Ryan, editors (McMaster Centre for Gerontological Studies, 2010).

Celebrating Poets Over 70

by Marianne Vespry

Celebrating Poets Over 70 began for me as an accidental project. I was feeling that I could and should move on after my husband's death. At a Tower Poetry meeting, Ellen Ryan described her vision of an elder-anthology, and then asked if I would edit it. Of course I don't step into such commitments blindly: I ask myself, "Why not?" and allow at least 10 seconds to pass to see if any compelling negatives present themselves. Nothing. I said "Yes."

Over the next months we received 1,100 poems, and with the help of 16 reader/evaluators, we winnowed them down to 330. We had decided to group the poems by themes, but we could not slot them into pre-set categories; we had no preexisting list of chapters. Rather I dealt them into piles of poems I hoped would illuminate each other. If a pile was too big, it was divided. If it was too small, it disappeared, and the poems were distributed among other piles. Twelve piles emerged, twelve piles in need of one-word titles. Sometimes it was easy: Childhood, Love, Death. Sometimes it was difficult: Encounters, Reflection.

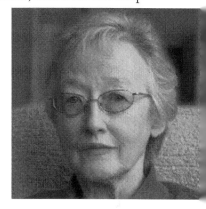

At the beginning it seemed so tenuous: Every poem records an Encounter, embodies its author's Reflections; all poetry is about Love and Death. But as each theme was sub-sorted, as each poem fell into place (fell or was pushed), the themes and even the placement on the page acquired inevitability. In the Introduction I apologized in advance to anyone who might feel that their poem was misplaced, but no one complained.

Individual themes offered surprises.

Childhood poems did not overflow with the innocence and optimism popular culture expects; they were mostly sober, even sad. Poets remembered dead siblings, a grandmother's funeral, the struggles of the immigrant experience, and the 1930s. The birth of a baby is wonderful:

>   this is the kind of news
>   that can set the tilting world
>   up straight.
>   — "Bret Andrew, February 5, 2003"
>   by Marion Frahm Tincknell

But another poet has a bleaker view; he sees the newborn as:

> a baby critter
> that didn't beg
> to be begotten
> on a hopeless
> starving stage
>   — "Basic Needs" by Jerry Andringa

Generations weaves together love, memory, recognition, concern, playfulness, the heartache and laughter that dance together through family interactions. A great-grandmother worries about her daughter, squeezed by sandwich generation obligations. The family traditions that chafed a child are now upheld by her much older self, and imparted in turn to her grandchildren. The Depression scarred and terrified a generation; the next generation deals with the fallout.

> After her mother moved to a nursing home
> Hazel cleared out her house.
> In a kitchen cupboard she found a jar labeled
> string too short for anything.
>   — "Saving" by Sharon MacFarlane

History starts with a tongue-in-cheek capsule biography of Julius Caesar, and a meditation on falconry.

>   Everything flows,
>   says the old dark wisdom.
>   Blood flows, tears flow,
>   falcons are flown.

> — "Falcons and Their Kings"
> by Francis Sparshot

It goes on through more recent tragedies. Canada lost perhaps 100,000 marriageable young men in World War I, dead or severely wounded. That left an equal number of young women unmarried or widowed and unlikely to remarry. One of them writes:

> I never met the man
> I would have loved
> For in any war
> There is
> No rhyme
> No reason.
> — "Unknown" by Joan S. Nist

Love poems celebrate present love, recall beginnings, dream past loves back to us. A poet marvels at his good fortune:

> Your spirit is my flag freshly unfurled.
> Old Valentine! How new you make my world!
> — "Old Valentine" by Irving Leos

Another speaks of union and separation:

> till we peel
> limb by limb
> he from me
> me from him
> each to reach
> best we may
> separate selves
> born of the day
> — "One and One Are One" by Sandy Wicker

Another remembers:

> . . . long journeys
> Through the seas
> Of the mind, in
> A white ship, steered
> By the stars.

> Your hair
> Blowing in the wind.
> — "Under an Opal Moon" by Stephen Threlkeld

Encounters spills forth with rich moments and seasons of life.

> In a well-loved house,
> ...the ghosts
> of former tenants...
> ...whisper from the rooms and on the lawn
> but leases end and then we, too, are gone.
> — "Passing Through" by Patricia Brodie

> Emigrants are forever divided from those they left in "the old country":
> we travel through
> each others' lives
> only in thought
> we left our souls behind
> by leaving
> — "Emigrants" by Giselle Braeuel

> At a summer music festival in Ottawa, a concertgoer muses about post-9/11 security in the U.S., preferring local arrangements:
> As for police sharpshooters here, or razor wire
> forget it: we have retained
> Beethoven, Mozart, Dvorak
> to provide our security.
> — "Security" by Christopher Levenson

The flavour of ***Aging*** is bittersweet. Losses are acknowledged, but what is left is valued even more. A poet says of her chimney sweep:

> He wears the leer of men who peer up more
> than sooty shafts. I pay no mind, for like the hearth,
> I know: when we no longer burn, we die.
> — "Chimney Sweep, November" by Elisavietta Ritchie

Moving out of the family home has been hard; the treasures stored in the attic have gone to family members who will value them.
> The attic is bare
> but my heart is full
> of what has been.
> — "Change" by Naomi C. Wingfield

New technology can help enrich old lives, substitute for failing senses:
> At one hundred
> Etta is au courant.
> Her watch talks to her.
> It is eleven fifteen.
> — "Lifetime" by Carrie McLeod Howson

Sometimes only the poet's skill is left to celebrate:
> Yesterday I was indestructible
> eighteen, the sea
> was deep; today
> decaying in the shallows.
> — "Macular Degeneration"
> by Killian McDonnell

Who would have expected the funny poems about **Death**? They share space with the elegiac:
> And the long snows of winter
> Softly settle upon them all.
> — "Farewell to Friends" by Joan Shewchun

> ...and afterwards [we]
> talked incessantly, unwilling
> to finally confront the silence
> of her loss.
> — "Celebrations" by Don Gralen

and the refusal to "go gentle":
> I'll be like that leaf,
> hang on to that damn

limb no matter how hard
the gusts whip me around.
— "Obstinance" by Nancy Gotter Gates

The part on **Nature** begins with three poems about deer and goes on to water: water birds, living by the water. Next are the seasons.

winter: Champagne air, dry, biting,
dances with light.
Wind-scoured snow, trackless,
flashes with diamond fire.
— "–50C" by Isobel Spence

spring: rain-drenched tulips
my inside out
umbrella
— "Haiku: Tulips" by Sonja Dunn

summer: The wasps are in the windfalls,
Take care, my dear, don't touch!
— "Late Summer Warning"
by Muriel Jarvis Ackinclose

fall: The last leaf to fall
sees on its earthbound spiral
the first buds of spring
— "Season Haiku" by Julie Adamson

Reflections serves up memories, dreams, arguments, meditations, wisdom. Sometimes the reflections are literal:

I can reflect back the sunshine's bright beams,
recovering sky-tinted shards of my dreams.
— "Shards of Glass" by Marion Wyllie (age 103)

Sometimes being mindful is hard to bear:

> The pot simmers, I stir, taste, season.
> A roadside bomb kills an American soldier
> and two Iraqis . . .
> — "Mindful Soup" by Sylvia Levinson

Reading obituaries, a poet thinks about her own:
> Loved ones, when you write my obituary,
> say this: Once, sitting still,
> she turned into a tiger.
> — "Reading Obituaries" by Mildred Tremblay

Sometimes poetry itself is a path to wisdom:
> The Advocate
> stopped playing god
> The Pacifist fought
> to find inner peace
> And the old Survivor
> healed her wounds with words.
> — "Getting There" by Lorna Louise Bell

Dementia — There are funny poems about death, but no one can make light of dementia.
> . . . it takes and takes and takes
> until all that's left is one working heart,
> locked inside a warm empty body
> that's forgotten how to die.
> — "Morning Musing" by Diane Buchanan

Memory — Poetry arises out of memory. Wordsworth said that it "… takes its origin from emotion recollected in tranquility." "Memory" as a specific theme might appear redundant, until you read the poems. They talk of remembering and forgetting (accidental and deliberate), of voices and silences and ghosts from the past.
> I heard the wind in the night
> And I remembered.
> — "Memory" by Isobel Spence

Words celebrates language, writing, poetry:
> I read poetry
> and for a short time
> live inside a stranger's world
>> — "I am the Poet of My Courtyard" by Rita Katz

It celebrates communication and its failures:
> Please
> relax
> listen
> slide into reverie
> linger with me
>> — "They Say, I Say" by Joyce Harries

And indeed, it celebrates words:
> I love friends and flowers and birds
> I must add, I do love words!
>> — "I Love Words" by Marion Wyllie (age 103)

Invitations to Practice

WRITING AND AGING WITH SPIRIT
by Ellen S. Jaffe

My mother, Viola, wrote these lines at age 90, in her room at an assisted living residence. She had always written "light verse" for family occasions but started writing poetry seriously, as a way of expressing and voicing her feelings, when she entered the residence at age 89. She wrote until the end of her life at 91 — in her words: "Something occurs, I react, and a poem results. Feelings turn into language, and language validates my feelings." I think that she wrote to better understand herself and the world around her, and to find a way through the world's mystery, chaos, and silence. Even — or especially — at that time in her life, writing helped her on her spiritual journey, helped her define her place in the world and in relationship to others. After one of her tablemates died (a not-uncommon occurrence in residences and nursing homes), she wrote,

Lonely or Alone
(Excerpt)

I sit here day after day
Alone but not lonely...
I've learned to be alone,
I'll never learn to be lonely.
— Viola Jaffe

> One more death, an empty chair at the table,
> No one cares, no one marks the passing,
> Each one thinks, "Who's next? Not I, not I."
> One death as important as 300 in Pakistan, thousands in Darfur.
> One person less, but a person, a woman I knew.

My mother was still alert, able to watch and care about the news as she had done all her life; she was aware of death on a large scale, far away, publicized in the media — but she was also able to see and mourn the death of one person, her friend, even when other residents and staff kept silent.

Writing allows us to do this: to bear witness to ourselves, our loved ones, and the world.

Why Write?

We often turn to writing and other art forms at turning points in life — adolescence and sexual flowering, love, birth of children and grandchildren, illness, loss and grief, growing old. We find words and images (my love is like a red red rose; her icy heart) for our deepest, most joyful, or devastating feelings, and this can help us go through these times without getting so lost. Poetry and other writing helps us to empathize with the feelings of others and also to feel we are less alone in our own feelings; many people have found poems or quotes that are healing in times of grief or which express the ecstasy of love. As we age, we tend to look both backwards and forwards, and also to see the present with new eyes — and writing can help us come to terms with the self we are now becoming. Finding the "right" word or combination of words can be a kind of "open sesame" to the treasure trove of understanding.

The word we use about the process of aging is interesting in itself. We talk about "growing" old — which implies we are still growing, like a tree, or the grass, or the gardens we have tended all our lives. We may be growing in different ways, but we are still growing, we continue to grow — to flower, to fruit, to change, to go on. The word "grow" is related to "green" — the color of new grass and leaves. The green chlorophyll in plants is what allows them to turn sunlight into food and energy, the process of photosynthesis. How can we, metaphorically, keep this chemical/physical process alive in ourselves as long as we can? We need to be careful not to shut the door on this spiritual and emotional growth — and then accept the burst of color, the sweet fruit, as the green fades.

Your writing need not be for publication, and certainly should not start out that way. You are developing a relationship with yourself, with the hidden corners of your mind; you are exploring that dark basement, that attic full of old suitcases, those birds flying just outside your window, and your own (sometimes unfamiliar) body. Writing can become a practice — not in order to get "better" at it (though that will happen), but as a spiritual practice, a way to develop inner guides and guidelines, something that becomes part of your life.

How to Begin?

The first step is to find a journal or notebook that suits you, one that feels comfortable to write in — it might have a fancy cover or be a school exercise book. But it is important to have a book, rather than a collection of scattered papers that can disappear. You can paste a favorite photograph or art card on the cover if you like, to make it more personal.

It also sometimes helps to have a time to write — early morning, with tea after lunch, just before bed — whatever time suits you. But you also want to have the book at hand for thoughts and impressions that come spontaneously; you might see a beautiful rainbow, or have a wish for a loved person, or remember your mother's Aunt Clara and the cookies she baked for you, or suddenly recall your experiences as an immigrant child in a new school. Some people do write (or rewrite/copy and file) on the computer, and this is okay, but not necessary: Even writers who often use computers find it is good to have the physical experience of writing by hand — and a notebook is much more portable, user-friendly, and doesn't need batteries or electricity. You are your own source of power!

Journal entries can take the form of random paragraphs, a memoir, "letters" that you won't send but address to a particular person (even someone who has died — this is a wonderful way to still communicate in your mind and perhaps resolve some loose ends), poems (rhyming or just free verse), a piece of fiction (short story), or anything you like. You may have dabbled in writing earlier in your life — or not; now is the time to begin. It's possible you will want to meet with a group of friends (whether you live in your own home or in a retirement home or residence), to write together and, if you like, share your writing with each other, reading it aloud. Meeting regularly as a group (e.g., once a week, twice a month, etc.) helps one to focus, and when everyone does their own version of the same theme, surprising things can happen. The group need not be large — 4 to 6 people is a good size.

People often think they don't have time in their busy lives to write — or the prospect of looking at a blank page for hours, waiting to be inspired, is too daunting. One great way to overcome both these problems is to do a "timed writing" of 5 or 10 minutes (you can even start with 3 minutes — use an egg-timer!). The rule is to keep your hand moving for all that time. If you get stuck, you can simply repeat your title or subject, and then see what new words or ideas come. You can write a surprising amount in this time — and you may surprise yourself with the thoughts, images, and associations that come to mind in this "sprint" of energetic writing. Although in everyday life, we worry about our words making sense, following rational logic, and being useful to other people, in creative writing we are using the same words with a different purpose — to find images for our thoughts and feelings, to explore the past, to play with language, and to use our imagination, to dream, to wonder. Like Alice in Wonderland, we can become "curiouser and curiouser" about ourselves and the world around us.

A Few Exercises to Get Started

I will now suggest a few exercises to help you get started. These can be done on your own or in a group. They can be found in my book, *Writing Your Way: Creating a Personal Journal* (Toronto: Sumach Press, 2001). Information on ordering the book can be found at the end of this article.

> **1. Colors of My Mind** — The world around us is full of colors, to which we have our own associations. These can be personal, or cultural; the colors of weddings and mourning vary around the world. A color can suggest something in the outside world — red could make you think of a cardinal, or of your favorite sweater, for example — or a feeling, like love or anger. A color might even suggest a sound, or a smell. Write down a color (start with one you really like, then do one you dislike), and describe what each color makes you think of. There are two ways of doing this:
>
>> List at least four things each color makes you think of. These can be anything at all. Example: Blue: forget-me-nots, blue jays in the garden, my son's old baby blanket, Bessie Smith singing the blues.
>>
>> List your five senses (sight, hearing, smell, taste, touch) plus "emotion" and then write one or more associations to the color

you've chosen. Example: Red is the sight of a rose in bloom, the sound of a cardinal singing, the smell of fresh strawberries, the taste of hot peppers, the touch of velvet, the emotion of love, or of anger. The sense-images don't have to relate to objects having that color: for example, red could be "the sound of cymbals clashing," yellow could be "the sound of a child laughing." In both forms of the exercise, the more details you use, the better.

The exercise using the five senses can be used with other nouns: home; spring; holidays like Christmas, Passover, Ramadan, etc.

2. Body Language — One way of getting to know your own body is to write as if a part of your body is speaking: perhaps your hands, your hair, your eyes, your back, your feet. It can be an inner organ like the heart; it can even be a part of the body that is missing (either from birth or because of surgery, illness, or accident). Do a timed writing of 15 minutes. Before you start writing, take three deep breaths, relax your body in a way that feels comfortable to you, and see if you can hear the voice of a particular body part. It may be something you and others can see (hair, feet, breasts), or an organ deep inside. It may be an area where you have been experiencing illness, pain, or loss. You might try writing several pieces about different areas of your body, including parts you like as well as those you don't like or those that are causing you concern. The writing can be a series of paragraphs, a poem, a letter from your body part to you, or a dialogue between the two of you.

3. I remember/I don't remember — I learned this exercise from Natalie Goldberg's inspiring book *Writing Down the Bones*. Natalie also emphasizes the importance of timed writing, especially for this exercise. Write "I remember" on your paper, and for five minutes, write what you remember — you may find yourself focusing on a particular person or subject, or just writing at random (both are okay). If you feel stuck, go back to "I remember."

Read over what you've written. Then (now or next day), write the heading "I don't remember." *Wait, you're saying — how can I write about what I don't remember?* It's a paradox, but most of us know that there are things we can't remember — whether it is what we ate for breakfast yesterday, next week's doctor's appointment, or the house we lived in when we were 6 years old. Write about that. ("I don't remember the house in Albuquerque, New Mexico, but I know my mother always wanted to go back there…") You can even write something like "I don't remember a time when I wasn't called fat…," as one woman did in a workshop. If you are really ambitious, or curious, you can try writing this part of the exercise with your non-dominant hand: Sometimes this brings up deep memories. (Be prepared — but know that you only remember what you are able to handle.)

You are writing this for yourself, of course, but some of these memories may turn into memoirs or stories you can pass on to your children, grandchildren, and other family members.

4. Final Exercise — The late U.S. poet Audre Lorde wrote, "I am not only a casualty, I am also a warrior." How does this apply to your life?

Good luck! As novelist Ann Beatty says, "It is only through writing that you discover what you know." Another writer, Ali Smith, gives us this lovely image: "And it was always the stories that needed the telling that gave us the rope we could cross any river with. They balanced us high above any crevasse. They made us natural acrobats. They made us brave. They made us well. …." (from *Girl Meets Boy*).

Part III

Serving from Spirit

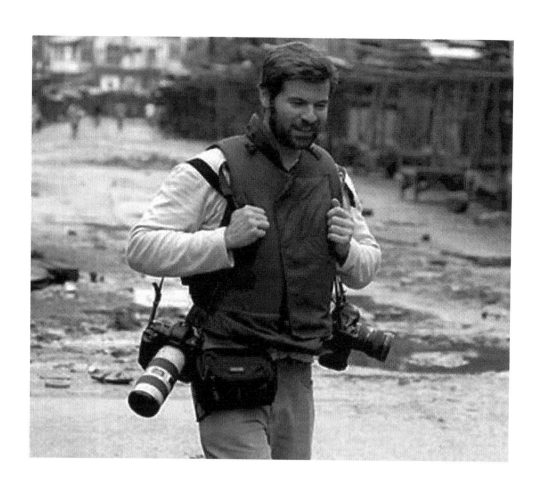

Remembering Christopher
by Bolton Anthony

When we lived in Fayetteville, North Carolina, during the mid-1970s, my oldest son, Edward, was friends with a boy who lived a block away and was a year and a half younger than he was. They were inseparable companions — "best buddies"— for six years. Then, when Edward was 12, we moved to Greensboro; and though we made the 90-mile journey back to Fayetteville once or twice a year, absent the vital, almost daily contact that sustains childhood camaraderie, their friendship languished.

Over the years, my wife stayed in contact with Christopher's mother; and we were aware how, as both our sons matured, a similar passion for photography — nascent during their childhood years — shaped and determined their later career choices.

Christopher was a stringer for the local newspaper, *The Fayetteville Observer*, while he was still in high school. At North Carolina State University, he worked on the campus newspaper, *The Technician*; then, after a master's degree from Ohio University, he returned home to work again for *The Observer*, this time as a staff photographer.

Then, in 1998, some strange attractor deflected the trajectory of his life away from what had, until then, been a predictable course. He moved to New York City and from that base honed his photojournalistic skills in all the major conflict zones of the past dozen years: Kosovo, Angola, Sierra Leone, Afghanistan, Kashmir, the West Bank, Iraq, and Liberia. Following September 11, he took photos at Ground Zero, then later covered the aftermath of Hurricane Katrina and the earthquake in Haiti.

His photographs appeared on the covers of *Newsweek* and *The Economist*, and on the front pages of *The New York Times*, *The Washington Post*, and the *Los Angeles Times*. His work was nominated for a Pulitzer Prize and honored with numerous other awards.[1]

On April 20, 2011, Chris Hondros was killed — along with fellow photojournalist Tim Hetherington — by a rocket-propelled grenade in Misrata, Libya, where he was covering the Libyan civil war. He was 41.

His friend, Greg Campbell, shared this on hearing of his death:

We talked about this special breed of journalism he was drawn to and how important it was to bear witness to atrocities that take place far from most of the world's eyes. He believed entirely in the power of photojournalism to change the world, to enlighten hearts and minds, and to bring justice and possibly comfort to those who are suffering the most. His deepest commitment, from the very beginning, was to honor those he photographed and bear witness to their struggles.[2]

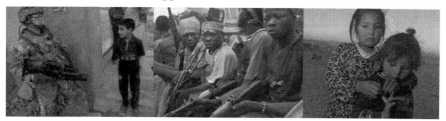

Chris Hondros was the product of the great American melting pot. His mother, Inge, had been born in 1936 in that part of eastern Germany which Poland annexed in 1946. His father, after whom he was named, had been born in Greece. His parents, child refugees after World War II, had met and married in New York. They moved to Fayetteville shortly after he was born, and he grew up in a large house and extended family that included his father's Greek parents and his younger brother Denos.

Everyone's life traces back to the mysterious, always improbable, intersection of two other lives. This is true whether your parents first met on the playground in pre-school or — like Chris's — were war-weary refugees washed ashore from the chaos of distant lands and forced to negotiate the intimate commerce of their shared daily life in a language that was alien to both. The embryo bursts forth from this fusion of two lives. To put the metaphor to further use: Perhaps, like its nuclear counterpart, the fusion creates a cache of latent energy.

When viewed from outside, Chris's life for its first 28 years seems to move within a predictable orbit. Then, at the point of inflection, a firewall is breached and the latent energy is unleashed. In the 13 years that follow, the distance he travels away from the immigrant Greek community of restaurateurs and shopkeepers of his childhood in Fayetteville rivals the distance his mother and father traveled in the journey to his conception.

How does one explain this? How does one account for those uncommon few among us who — in dramatic and undramatic ways — seeing wrong, are stirred to try to right it; seeing suffering, try to heal it; seeing war, try to stop it?[3] How does one account for the young civil rights activists who — a generation earlier — rode interstate buses into the segregated South, for the leavening of college graduates who gave two years of their lives to Peace Corps service, for the conscientious objectors who protested the violence of the Vietnam War? How does one account for those who cannot do what most of us usually manage well enough: just see *facts* flat on, without some horrible moral squint?[4]

Those were the questions I pondered at Chris's funeral, where I joined my son Edward and my daughter Shannon. The trajectory of his life had come full circle, ending here in a packed Greek Orthodox Church located not two blocks from his childhood home. The Greek community that filled the church to overflowing was the familiar community of his childhood and youth. My daughter, who in recent years had reconnected with Chris and visited him in New York, had an answer for my questions: "It was Inge," she told me; and she sent me something Chris had written:

> I grew up hearing tales of war from my mother… the sounds of American bombers flying over her village; the feelings of hunger when food ran short; the sight of her older brother Herbert in uniform and sent off to fight the Russians, [a cipher in the] columns of German troops marching east in tight formations, and returning west bedraggled and doomed after months on the front. [Then, during] the summer of 1946… all the ethnic Germans like my mother [who was 10] were forcibly expelled from the eastern fringe of Germany by revenge-minded Polish troops, who then annexed the lands…
>
> So when I started covering war as a journalist, she understood what was driving me better than many mothers might. When I showed her pictures of Kosovo refugees packed onto rusty trains, she nodded knowingly and related her own similar experiences. Tales of barbarity from Iraq elicited from her not empty platitudes, but informed observations of how easily stable societies can come unglued, and how quickly the horrific can become commonplace. My mother, like me, sees war as an abomination, but not an aberration; she has no expectations that humanity can ever fully escape the call to arms. We will probably always fight wars, but if we do we should

know what war means. Fulfilling that mandate is my main mission as a war photographer.[5]

Probably, there are no universal answers to the questions that gnawed at me. What kindles our compassion and spurs us — often against our own narrow self-interest — to act for the sake of another is always a part of our own unique story. Why this movement of grace happens in some lives and not others is shrouded in mystery.

But some lives do shine, some lives do sparkle. More than others. And Chris Hondros lived such a life. In his autobiography, *Report to Greco*, the great Greek writer, Nikos Kazantzakis, explains his motive for writing. As you read the words, substitute photography for writing and perhaps you will have a small window into Chris's soul:

> The more I wrote the more deeply I felt that in writing I was struggling, not for beauty, but for deliverance. Unlike a true writer, I could not gain pleasure from turning an ornate phrase or matching a sonorous rhyme; I was a man struggling and in pain, a man seeking deliverance. I wanted to be delivered from my own inner darkness and to turn it into light, from the terrible bellowing ancestors in me and to turn them into human beings.[6]

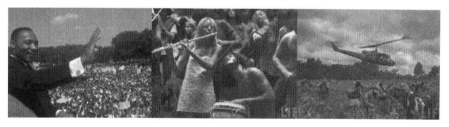

These ruminations have been informed in part by the news I received in early July, a month after Chris's funeral: Theodore Roszak — a social critic and cultural historian of the first rank, whose seminal book, *The Making of a Counter Culture: Reflections on the Technocratic Society*, helped define the generation that came of age during the tumultuous 60s — had died at his home in Berkeley, California, at age 77.

Though Ted went on to write some 20 books — including notably *The Voice of the Earth: An Exploration of Ecopsychology* (a field of inquiry he pioneered) and seven novels — most of the tributes published after his death focus on his early book which:

> ... offered a rationale for the so-called Summer of Love in 1967 and the eruption of student dissent a year later. He warned middle Americans that their greatest enemy lay not in Red China or Moscow but "sat facing them across the breakfast table." Roszak's thesis held that technology and the pursuit of science... had alienated the young. Consequently they sought comfort and "meaning" in psychedelic drugs, exotic religions and alternative ways of living.
>
> His "counterculture" neologism defined this "alternative society." Its members, he said, were long-haired young people, many smoking dope or dropping acid, listening to psychedelic rock or protest songs by Bob Dylan and Leonard Cohen. When they gathered at pop festivals, "love-ins," or student demonstrations, their concerns ranged from racial discrimination to global poverty and included what are now called "green issues."[7]
>
> The book argued that science-dominated modern society was ugly, repressive and soulless; that youthful dissent was coherent enough to be termed a culture; and that this anti-rationalist "counterculture"... might offer the foundation of a new visionary civilization.[8]

Few of the tributes mention the book that was the occasion for my working with Ted. He had called me during the summer of 2007 with a novel proposal. He had completed the manuscript of a book and then been frustrated by a long and futile search for a publisher. He thought of the new book, *The Making of an Elder Culture,* as a kind of sequel to the earlier book. "Boomers don't read," he had been told by would-be publishers, "and even if they did, they wouldn't read books about aging." He asked if Second Journey wished to publish the book online.

After a 40-year hiatus, Ted had returned to the boomers because he believed there was for "America's most audacious generation" a second act: In the "elder insurgency" Ted imagined, what the "boomers left undone in their youth, they will return to take up in their maturity."[9] In its youth, the boomer generation had discovered "the politics of consciousness transformation. 'You say you want a revolution... Well, you know, we all want to change your head.'" In its elder years Roszak believed it would perceive that:

Aging changes consciousness more surely than any narcotic; it does so gradually and organically. It digests the experience of a lifetime and makes us different people — sometimes so different that we are amazed, embarrassed, or even ashamed at the person we once were. Pious people often claim that religion offered them the chance to be born again. But, curiously enough, growing old can also lead to rebirth, a chance to leave old values, old obsessions, old fears, and old loves behind. Aging grants permission. It allows us to get beyond the assumptions and ambitions that imprisoned us in youth and middle age. That can be a liberating realization. Perhaps there is a biological impulse behind that possibility, a driving desire to find meaning in our existence that grows stronger as we approach death. It may even lead to rebellion, if one has the time and energy to undertake the act.[10]

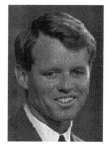 Think of the gift of "all those extra years of life," he urged us — the nearly 30 years of extended life expectancy that medical science and improvements in public health have over the past century created — think of them as a resource: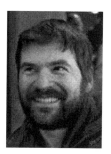

...a cultural and spiritual resource reclaimed from death in the same way the Dutch reclaim fertile land from the waste of the sea. During any one of those years, somebody who no longer has to worry about raising a family, pleasing a boss, or earning more money will have the *chance to join with others in building a compassionate society* where people can think deep thoughts, create beauty, study nature, teach the young, worship what they hold sacred, and care for one another.[11]

"You say you want a revolution?" Joining "with others in building a compassionate society" — now there's a revolution worth the making!

My recommendation is *The Spirit Level: Why Greater Equality Makes Societies Stronger* by Wilkinson and Pickett, a pair of English academics. Ironically, the title does not refer to spirituality, but to a carpenter's level, which is called a spirit level in England. But nonetheless, I take my definition of spirituality from Abraham Heschel, the rabbi who marched with Martin Luther King: Abraham Heschel called spirituality the ecstatic force that stirs all our goals. *The Spirit Level* does that for me. It tells us of the central importance of wealth equality — a concept that is one of the boldest, most exciting ideas of our time. The book gathers research that shows how inequality destroys a society. For instance, it shortens all of our lives — lives of the rich as well as the poor. As wealth inequality goes up, so does violence, mental illness, unhappiness, imprisonment, and even teenage pregnancy and obesity! Ultimately it threatens democracy and the well-being of the people. This idea, for me, has become an ecstatic force that stirs all my goals.

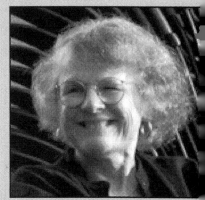

Cecile Andrews

Cecile Andrews' work has been featured in the videos "Escape from Affluenza" (PBS) and "Consumed by Consumption" (TBS) and in *The New York Times, Los Angeles Times, Esquire*, and various PBS and NPR programs. She is the author of *Slow Is Beautiful: New Visions of Community, Leisure and Joie de Vivre,* and *The Circle of Simplicity: Return to the Good Life* and the co-editor, with Wanda Urbanska, of *Less is More: Embracing Simplicity for a Healthy Planet, a Caring Economy and Lasting Happiness*. A former community college administrator, Cecile has been a visiting scholar at Stanford University and affiliated scholar at Seattle University. Visit her Web site at at www.cecileandrews.com.

I Don't Do Old

there are things to do,
lilies to grow.
Stella d'ore's blooms
are my galaxy.
irises' blue . . . fill
my eyes with
ecstasy,
i don't do old
i do global warming
with Suzuki, Schindler
and Al Gore's concern
with climates
in crisis.
my affinity is with
the arctic — ice, melt, water,
polar bears
drowning —
i don't do old.
god's creativity,
and ideas light
my spirit.

art, literature
can fill me
with awe.
life is sweet,
never, i will
never age out,
i don't do old.
kindness spins
my web,
altruism, a.i.d.s, h.i.v.,
world poverty
are my bonds . . .
entanglements of
laughter are the gossamer
threads that
tie my connections together . . .
i won't do old

— sterling haynes[†]

[†] Published in *Celebrating Poets over 70*, M. Vespry and E. Ryan, editors (McMaster Centre for Gerontological Studies, 2010).

PEACE THROUGH PEACEFUL MEANS

by Betsy Crites

I dimly remember that day in late August, 1963, when my parents and I walked across Memorial Bridge to join the March on Washington for Jobs and Freedom. We had just moved to the Northern Virginia suburbs the year before. I was 12 and still homesick for the farm in Colorado where I'd grown up, so more than anything I remember the crowds — I'd never seen so many people together. I later learned, neither had anyone else.

Now in my 60s, I look back and marvel at how Dr. Martin Luther King, Jr., and the civil rights movement set the direction for my life. Not only did they bring together 250,000 people — the largest peaceful gathering the country had seen up to that time — but more importantly, their nonviolent methods and example allowed all of us working for a more just and peaceful society to expand what we thought possible. We know now that large-scale social progress can be accomplished through peaceful means. In fact, it is the only way to achieve such progress.

As I plumb the depths of nonviolence, I've also learned that its power goes beyond effective strategy for social movements. It can also effect profound changes at the individual level. The discoveries of Dr. King, Mohandas Gandhi, and many others going back to the Buddha and Jesus have shaped my journey as a peace activist and guided my aspirations to be a person of peace.

The seeds of my activism planted that day on the Washington Mall grew in the direction of U.S. international relations, peace, and nonviolence. I was a student in Peru in 1970 and later joined the Peace Corps in Honduras. A few years later my husband and I returned to Guatemala where I worked as a health educator. These were particularly volatile times in Central America. Witnessing the impact of

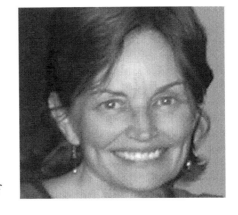

U.S. economic and military intervention became the frame for my understanding of the violence that consumed the region for the next decade and beyond.

We returned to the U.S. in 1981 so that I could pursue my Master's in public health. As soon as I finished my degree, however, my attention turned back to Central America.

The rising tide of violence during the 1980s that swept the very countries where we'd lived tore at my heart. President Reagan thought he saw the specter of communism spreading from Central America all the way to Texas. His response was to direct the CIA to arm and train the Nicaraguan contras and to send military aid to the brutal military regimes of El Salvador and Guatemala.

There was some truth in the CIA's intelligence. Many of the revolutionaries in Central America were influenced by Marx; some believed in a collective economy, some were armed, and some went to Cuba for training. But most people fighting in Central America, with or without guns, were responding to the extreme disparities in wealth, the oppression of poverty, and worst of all, the violent repression of military dictatorships. For the vast majority, the poles of communism and capitalism were meaningless abstractions.

Unfortunately, the President greatly oversimplified the problems and exaggerated the threat to the U.S. Consequently, U.S. military and economic policies caused immense unnecessary suffering and death.

As with most public discourse in America, this conflict in Central America became polarized. I know that I avoided ever mentioning the presence of Marxist revolutionaries, so as not to trigger the fears and distortions that were endemic to the Cold War period. Some discourse was just too emotionally charged to touch.

In hindsight, I know I might have approached this challenge with a spirit of truth seeking, spoken out of my own experience, and acknowledged dispassionately whatever piece of the truth emerged from the opposition. This is no easy task; our media thrives on controversy, and the system is set up as a competition between adversaries. As a society we value winning above truth and perception above reality. Our painful divisions leave us immersed in a battle of wills and all too often, in the international arena, in a battle of militaries.

One of the most difficult things seems to be to hold one's point of view lightly, remain open to new information and to all points of view, and be rigorous in the search for truth. My contribution in the 80s would have been much more valuable had I fully appreciated this aspect of nonviolence.

When possible, nonviolent movements employ traditional methods with patience and persuasion. For most successful movements, however, there eventually comes a moment, a tide when "taken at the flood" leads to a major shift in collective perception. It may be that historical conditions create the moment or the nonviolent actors may stimulate the conditions or a combination of both. Ideally, those actors will recognize the moment and step up their game.

In a highly charged and sometimes dangerous situation, nonviolent activists have an opportunity to draw upon their inner resources to call up voluntary sacrifices in hopes of pulling the parties into another level of "conversation." Gandhi described it this way: "Things of fundamental importance to the people are not secured by reason alone but have to be purchased with their suffering… if you want something really important to be done you must not merely satisfy the reason, you must move the heart also."

The risk comes because there is usually no way to predict the full range of the consequences. It is the willingness to expose oneself to harm — rather than inflict harm — that can change hearts. Many remember videoed scenes of police attacking Civil Rights activists with fire hoses and dogs. People were beaten and jailed, and the sight of this abuse shook the national conscience.

The effort which I became deeply involved in — Witness for Peace — was an experiment in this same tradition; personal risk and sacrifice were a way to awaken the awareness of wrongdoing.

In 1983, three dozen people of faith from North Carolina traveled to the Honduran/Nicaraguan border to witness personally

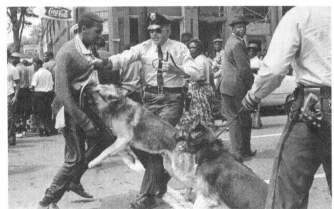

A young demonstrator is attacked by a police dog in Birmingham, AL, in May 1963. Scenes like these helped usher in the nation's landmark civil rights law, the 1965 Voting Rights Act. © Bill Hudson/AP

the impact of U.S. policy. Within weeks of their return they organized a second, larger group of 150 people from 32 states, to return to that border and continue providing a peaceful presence as a deterrent to violence. A few months later, Witness for Peace (WFP) was launched as a continuous presence that stood in defiance of the violence funded by our government.

For the next decade, I dedicated myself to that effort, coordinating the delegation program from the States, leading many delegations to Nicaragua and (after 1987) to Guatemala, and later serving as director of the national organization.

Over the next few years, thousands of U.S. citizens traveled to war-torn countries with all the dangers that entailed. The possibility of encountering violence or being subject to kidnapping was added to the challenges of the unfamiliar language, food, and culture. They returned with personal stories of the Nicaraguans and Guatemalans they had met and the destruction they saw being wrought with our tax dollars. They provided a powerful "witness" to their communities and to their Congressional representatives back home.

Was there a change in policy? Though the Reagan Administration lobbied intensely against our efforts, the pressure from returning WFP delegates and others prompted Congress in 1988 to prohibit future contra aid. By this point, however, the situation had become so polarized that the Administration went outside the law to continue funding the contras. Nevertheless, this is one of the rare occasions when the Congress did not give a President what he wanted in a time of foreign conflict. The strategy to provide a nonviolent presence and to convey the stories and testimonies of those people on the other end of U.S. policies won a significant advance.

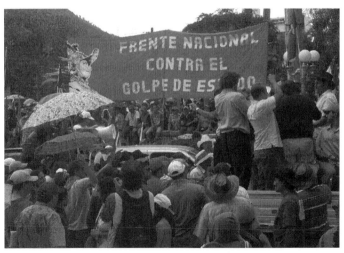

The troubled human rights conditions in Honduras continue. A June 2009 military coup provoked this protest. See witnessforpeace.org/section.php?id=132

Why did so many people volunteer to travel to a poverty-stricken region that had been ignored by the U.S. government and travel agents alike? Why I was doing it was clear. I had lived in Central America, had friends in danger, had a better than average understanding of the history and culture of the region, and had very deep sympathy for the people who were suffering extreme violence as a result of U.S. military and CIA interventions. I spoke Spanish and knew my way around these countries. Going into war zones added some risk, and I did have to face my fears about the uncertainties; but I knew I had competencies for managing potential problems.

For most people, however, the 2-week "delegation" required genuine courage. The trips to Nicaragua and Guatemala meant entering an unknown hostile environment at considerable expense and risk. WFP made clear in its two-day orientation that this would not be a vacation. We were going into zones of military conflict. In spite of that, people choose to "stand with" the Nicaraguan people suffering the effects of U.S. intervention. It somehow captured the imagination. Many people were outraged by the rhetoric they heard from the White House and inspired by the idealistic goals that the new government of Nicaragua seemed committed to. With this outrage came energy; we provided a constructive channel for that energy — a way for many people to act on their conscience.

In order to create a shift, the nonviolent activists may voluntarily endure hardships, injury, and even death to reopen a path to positive change. The Civil Rights movement, Witness for Peace, and many other organized efforts in nonviolence have broken unjust laws or otherwise exposed themselves to the fury of the opponent. They do this as a way to awaken the conscience of the adversary and interrupt the cycle of violence and/or awaken the public's awareness of problems.

Nonviolence does not promise quick and easy results; but it usually involves less injury, destruction, and loss of life, and it generally preserves space for constructive solutions.

A commitment to truth, a willingness to sacrifice, and many other insights and strategies have emerged from the history of nonviolent social change. Activists and scholars have learned some core principles which may overlap and interlock but are worth examining separately for the wisdom each brings forth. As more and more we integrate the principles of nonviolence into our thinking and our lives, the more we can open to the creative possibilities beyond force, and the more successful we activists will become in effecting long-term change.

The student of nonviolence could begin with these:

- **We all have a piece of the truth, but no one has all the truth.** As clear cut as things appear from our perspective, our opponents also believe they are right. Genuinely seeking the truth in the opponents' perspective helps us find some common ground and understand their worldview. This understanding can help us appeal to their higher nature or at least their particular interests.

- **Respect everyone.** The principle here is to avoid ever humiliating anyone *or* accepting humiliation from others. People sometimes change their minds, especially when given the space to do so. When harassed or disrespected, people defend and justify themselves to save face. Gandhi maintained friendly communications with the British Raj throughout his campaign to free India.

- **Never be against persons, be against problems.** This is related to the above principle and opens a way to respect the humanity of everyone without endorsing their behavior. We can oppose ideas, policies, and actions. We can deal at the level of problem solving, not name-calling. "The real success in nonviolence, which violence can never achieve, is to heal relationships. Even in a case of extreme violence, Gandhi felt it was possible to 'hate the sin, not the sinner.'"[1]

- **Set constructive strategic goals, but do not cling to the outcomes.** The vast web of cause and effect is constantly in flux, and it's impossible to know the full range of outcomes from any action. Dr. King wrote, "The beauty of nonviolence is that in its own way and in its own time it seeks to break the chain reaction of evil."[2] Through nonviolence we are better able to achieve some positive ends though it may not be what we originally envisioned. Our task is to stay grounded in our principles and flexible on nonessential details.

- **Recognize that means are ends in the making.** Showing respect, standing firm with the truth as we see it, and at times accepting adverse consequences or abuse without retaliation will stop and even reverse the cycle of violence. The purity of our motives

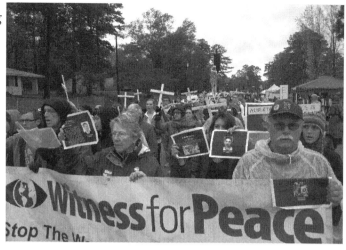

An annual vigil protesting the continued operation of the School for the Americas at Fort Benning, GA, where training is provided mainly to Latin American military officers, has occurred every November since 1990.

and the skill of our actions are critical and will have unforeseen positive spin-offs. The focus for any encounter is as much on the means as the ends.

- **Be prepared to sacrifice, but never intend to inflict harm.**
  When the adversary is unmoved and an unjust or violent situation persists, the activists need to, as Gandhi said, "not only speak to the head but move the heart also." The specter of civil rights protesters being attacked with fire hoses and dogs shook the conscience of the nation and, I believe, the attackers themselves.

As my understanding of these principles of nonviolence has grown, they have provided a measure I've used to gauge the efforts I want to support. A recent example is the current Forward Together (Moral Mondays) movement in North Carolina.

Moral Mondays emerged in the summer of 2013 in response to extreme measures taken by the N.C. state legislature, which had passed laws refusing federal funding for Medicaid and unemployment insurance; cut public school funding while at the same time expanding private schools; and increased obstacles to voting by the young, elderly, poor, and African American. These and many other policies seemed designed to favor wealthy, white constituents and reduce government by and for the people.

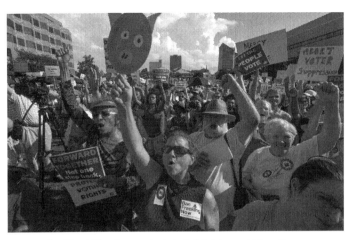

The Moral Mondays protests in Raleigh brought together a broad coalition of faith groups, civil rights groups, women's rights groups, immigration rights groups, and others.

The leadership of the state's NAACP seized this moment to lead a nonviolent response. Like many of my cohort who came of age in the sixties, I felt compelled to join this effort despite some personal risk and expense. I attended numerous rallies on the grassy mall outside the legislative building where gray heads peppered the crowd, and ultimately I joined those who risked arrest in order to make their voices heard.

As I've watched and participated in the Moral Monday process, I've been impressed with the leaders' faithfulness to the principles of nonviolence. They have carefully avoided personal attacks on the governor or legislators, keeping their focus on the harshness of the policies and the hardships they create. They emphasize respect for the police who arrested us. They set constructive goals such as registering voters.

For many who are taking part, whether it's through civil disobedience or volunteering in other ways, it is an act and leap of faith. We cannot know the outcomes of our efforts. Our faith is in the nonviolent means, which are developed and supported in a community of fellow activists.

In the strong tradition of the Civil Rights movement and Witness for Peace, Rev. William Barber and the other leaders of the Forward Together include prayer, reflection, and singing as a regular part of their gatherings. These are intentionally ecumenical. Though to some they might appear merely religious, they are deep practices that sew optimism and unity.

Time for reflection also tends to draw people back to the wisdom traditions that can inspire our highest motivations and purest intentions. The cultivation of peaceful attitudes such as gratitude, forgiveness, and compassion build the foundation for what Dr. King called the "beloved community," which can model the very ends it seeks to bring into being.

A specific book related to my spiritual journey — ah, choose. So many have come (and sometimes gone), as if one were a promiscuous lover surveying the past. *The Way of Zen* by Alan Watts was a first love. I was an alienated teenager stuck at a parents' party when I plucked it off a bookshelf. Suddenly, a world unfolded, so different from my own, yet striking a mystical chord that I didn't know was in me: Zen meditation and joyful Taoist masters, perplexing koans, sudden flashes of insights, a world of here and now Oneness that transcended all dualities, even that chasm between life and death.

I was launched on a journey that wound through countless authors and spiritual traditions: I recall with fondness *Autobiography of a Yogi* by Paramahansa Yogananda, *Play of Consciousness* by Swami Muktananda, *The Way of Man: According to the Teaching of Hasidism* by Martin Buber, *The Return of the Prodigal Son* by Henri Nouwen, and *God's Joyful Surprise* by Sue Monk Kidd and pretty much anything translated by Stephen Mitchell or Jonathan Star or written by Eknath Easwaran or Ram Dass. But wait, am I back to a promiscuous list of my many lovers?

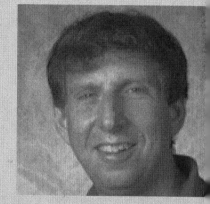

Drew Leder

Maybe "mentors" is a better term. Not only friends, teachers, bosses, and relatives can be our mentors, but the authors who grab us at just the right moment. Call them then "mo-mentors"? In that moment they give us momentum, and create a spiritual memento that can help us recall and return to our true self.

Drew Leder, M.D., Ph.D., is a professor of Philosophy at Loyola University Maryland, and the author of numerous articles and five books, including *Spiritual Passages: Embracing Life's Sacred Journey* (Tarcher, 1997), and *Sparks of the Divine: Finding Inspiration in our Everyday World* (Sorin, 2004). He gives talks and workshops around the country on creative aging. See http://evergreen.loyola.edu/dleder/www/.

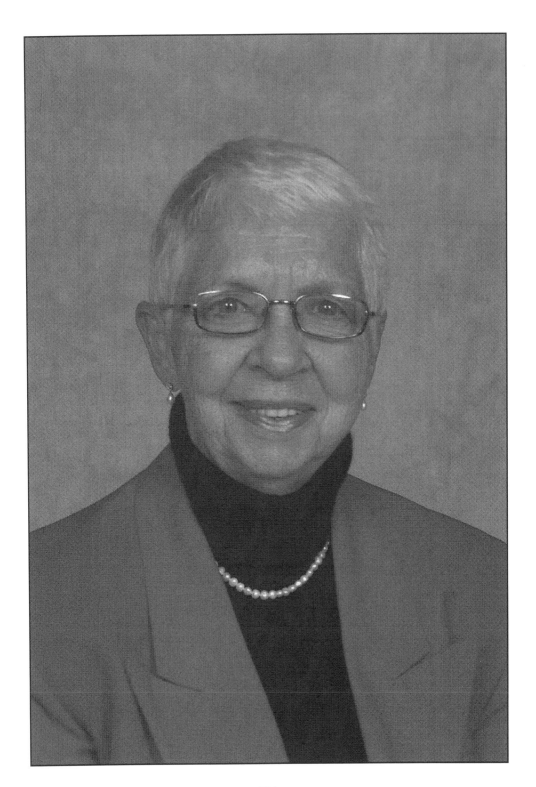

Honoring Our Elders

DENE PETERSON: THE SPRITE OF ELDERSPIRIT

> *My seventies were interesting and fairly serene, but my eighties are passionate. I grow more intense as I age.*
> — Florida Scott-Maxwell

These words aptly describe Dene Peterson, not in their particulars — she was passionate in her 70s! — but in their spirit. I remember seeing *Moulin Rouge* with her when she was but a spry 72. The movie about a poet in love with a cabaret actress/courtesan was sexual, rocking, flamboyant, and outrageous in its rapid-fire cinematography and cutting. It left me in the dust, but not Dene, who enjoyed it thoroughly. I couldn't have had a more fun date than with this ex-nun and distinguished elder.

In the Bible, Sarah is unexpectedly and repeatedly challenged by God. Uprooted from their home, she and Abraham must in their old age travel at God's whim to a new promised land. She, like Abraham, is given a new name (Sarai is changed to Sarah) and — at the ripe old age of 90 — informed that she is to have a child. Her reaction? She laughs. And when the prediction is miraculously fulfilled, she names her child "Isaac" — which means, in Hebrew, "to laugh."

Dene is Sarah, Sarah is Dene. How many times has she heeded God's call and moved to new places, assumed new identities, given birth to new projects and new versions of the self? Born in Kentucky, one of 11 children in an energetically Catholic family, at age 18 she became a Glenmary Sister. Dedicated to serving the poor and marginalized, she worked in Chicago… and Ohio… and Michigan — ever birthing new projects. Called to be a nun, she then experienced herself called out — along with the majority of Glenmary Sisters — to pursue their service work independent of the institutional hierarchy. When the age of "retirement" came, it became the moment for new birthing — her grandbaby being the ElderSpirit Community.

Though ElderSpirit upholds the traditional association of elderhood with wisdom and spirituality, overstating the radical nature of this experiment in communal living — and its importance — is difficult. ElderSpirit was the first senior cohousing community founded in the United States. It is also the first model of a residential setting where elders of all faith traditions (or none) can use their later years to support one another, serve social justice and the planet Earth, deepen their contemplative practice, and grow closer to God/Spirit.

In a land where aging can mean isolation — or self-centeredness — or institutionalization — Dene has shown us a different model. Dwelling just off the beautiful Virginia Creeper Trail, in Abingdon, Virginia, ElderSpirit residents own or rent their own homes — the community is resolutely mixed income — yet share common spaces to eat, meet, meditate, and worship. They are engaged in outward service and inward contemplation. They live together, age together, and maintain that support through illness, disability, and death.

Dene may be the Dean of ElderSpirit, but her gift has been to bring so many together — members of FOCIS (Federation of Communities in Service), co-leaders of the community, the Retirement Research Foundation, government agencies, prospective residents, and supporters — to make this "promised land" a reality.

Elderspirit Community now houses 40 residents. It has become a national model and a site for training communities around the country who wish to birth similar late-life experiments. She well deserves the Lifetime Achievement Award granted her at the 2011 National Cohousing Conference.

But what is her "lifetime achievement"? Herself? I know her as a person whose well-earned self-esteem is tempered with humility. "I am the first one to receive this award with but one project under their belt," she said at the Conference, "and I made lots of mistakes doing it." Mostly I think of Dene's delightful sense of humor. "At 50," wrote George Orwell, "everyone has the face he deserves." Dene has such a face, filled with "wrinkles" which are really smile-lines. She made me laugh that evening when, visiting ElderSpirit, I found myself spirited away to *Moulin Rouge*, an outrageous film made more enjoyable by the outrageous person by my side.

In the Bible, when Sarah named her child "Isaac" (to laugh), she explained, "God has brought me laughter; everyone who hears will laugh with me." Let us laugh with Dene at a lifetime of joy and service. Let us laugh at her "retirement," which was really a rebirth. Let us laugh at ElderSpirit Community, an impossible dream that now boasts some 29 completed homes.

If Dene's 70s and 80s are this passionate — who knows what's coming next?

— Drew Leder

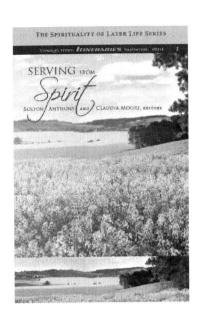

SERVING FROM SPIRIT

2011 Summer issue of Itineraries: Selections and Supplements

Pentecost with Andrew Harvey: Thoughts on Sacred Activism
    by Claudia Moore, Contributing Editor 139

What a Long, Strange Trip It's Been
    by Edith Kusnic. 145

How Can YOU Help?
    by Robert C. Atchley. 153

Healing the World
    by Judith Helburn 159

Jock Brandis: Championing Stone Age Technology
    by Pat and Steve Taylor 163

Pentecost with Andrew Harvey: Thoughts on Sacred Activism

by Claudia Moore

> *Everyone whose eyes are open knows the world is in a terrifying crisis. As many of us as possible need to undergo a massive transformation of consciousness and to find the sacred passion to act from this consciousness in every arena and on every level of reality.*
> — Andrew Harvey

OVER A LIFETIME, CERTAIN EVENTS blaze forth like beacons that mark turns on our path. For me, one such event took place on the Feast of the Pentecost, May 15, 2005. In search of the spark to rekindle the dry tinder of rote weekly religious worship, this particular morning I'd driven to a neighboring town where an alternative faith group met in a strip mall storefront "chapel" that had recently undergone its own conversion experience.

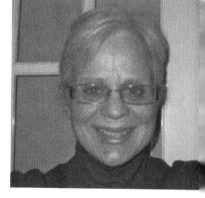

Unhappy about the status quo of my spiritual life, I knew that the heart of my discomfort was that I desired to serve Spirit, though I didn't know what that might mean. I had no clue of how exactly my request for clarity was about to be answered as I made my way into the building and found a seat. The roar of the enthusiastic welcome that greeted Andrew Harvey, the guest speaker that morning, suggested that something unusual was about to unfold.

For those unfamiliar with his life and work, Andrew Harvey is an internationally acclaimed poet, novelist, translator, mystical scholar, and spiritual teacher. Harvey has published over 20 books including *The Hope: A Guide to Sacred Activism* and *Heart Yoga: The Sacred Marriage of Yoga and Mysticism*. In addition to exploration and explication of Rumi and Sufi mysticism, he collaborated with Sogyal Rinpoche and Patrick Gaffney in the writing of *The Tibetan Book of Living and Dying*. Harvey was a Fellow of All Souls College, Oxford from 1972–1986 and has taught at Oxford University, Cornell University, The California Institute of Integral Studies, and the University of Creation Spirituality, as well as various spiritual centers throughout the United States. He was the subject of the

1993 BBC film documentary *The Making of a Modern Mystic*. He is the Founder of the Institute for Sacred Activism in Oak Park, Illinois, where he lives.

On that drear New England Sunday, Harvey began softly but quickly turned up the heat:[1]

> I'd like to share a practical vision with you of what being a mystical activist in a time like this really means. I beg you to listen — from my heart to your heart — because if you don't listen now, the crises that are coming will make it even harder to listen. It is extremely important to realize that we are not going to get out of this crisis… We will not avoid the bill for our monstrous shadow. We are going into storms that will shake humanity in unparalleled ways. Unless you and I are strong now, those storms will threaten us with madness and despair.
>
> The divine work I'm offering to you is not luxury. It's not something you can decide to do or not. It is something that if you hear what I'm trying to say to you on this day of Pentecost, you will realize it is something you have got to do to stay clear yourself and to be useful to others in any serious way at this moment. True prophets bring warnings and empowerments. And the Mother herself brings warnings and empowerments.
>
> There is no authentic spirituality in a time like this without a commitment to do something. You are the most privileged race that's ever been on the Earth. You belong to the most powerful nation on this Earth, which is responsible for a quarter of the emissions that are causing global warming and for a foreign policy that is hurtling the world towards Armageddon. It is time that we of the West wake up and claim our divinity, not just inwardly but in a conscious act of self-donation to making ourselves radioactive nuisances at a time when we have to turn up as real people or be guilty of the matricide of the planet.

Harvey closed the morning service with these words: "What is being asked of us by the Mother, by the flames, is that we stand in the middle of this apocalypse to see it for what it is, to see the birth and to know the birth in ourselves, to give ourselves over to the birth, and then, to stand in great passion and great joy, with great energy and give and give and give and serve and serve and serve and become, at last, truly authentic and truly divine."

Thunderous applause signaled the close of the service. Whoever this guy was, I knew without doubt that he spoke in tongues of fire. No longer a dusty Bible story, Pentecost had just become live in Technicolor for me. Reeling, I made my way to the table in the lobby where I bought a ticket for the afternoon workshop, which would delve more deeply and more practically into Harvey's concept of "Sacred Activism." As I sat in my car in the parking lot waiting for the doors to open once more, I remembered the adage, "Be careful what you wish for..." The irony that my prayer for a spirit-igniting spark was answered on that Pentecost in the form of a sacred activist wielding a blowtorch wasn't lost on me.

Over the course of the afternoon, Harvey outlined what we each must do to become sacred activists. As I listened, I thought about what had seemed to be a mysterious impetus that led me to return to college at age 50 to complete two degrees in social work. For an also unknown reason, I chose to specialize in community organization. Courses that focused on how to help people come to consensus, to strategize for empowerment, and to come to victory for the greater good somehow resonated deeply. Though unable to see an exact way I could use the education I'd acquired in combination with what might be described as eclectic life experience, after hearing Harvey's message, I sensed that soon enough, I'd find a way to live my service to Spirit as some sort of elder sacred activist.

However, along with this revelation, some significant questions took form. What does it mean to be an elder in a culture rife with ageism? What does it mean to be part of a demographic of people turning 65 at the rate of 8,000 per day? While I have no definitive answers to these questions, I have observations to offer based upon my experience working with elders and my experience of my own aging.

Not so long ago, I worked in an assisted living facility. Make that to read "warehouse-for-elders-who-don't-yet-require-full-nursing-care-but-their-families-for-some-reason-don't-want-them-at-home." The most difficult aspect of my job was to witness the effects of isolation and the sense of utter purposelessness so many of the residents voiced. These were men who had headed some of the biggest corporations in the country. These were women who ran hugely successful volunteer organizations. These were men and women who knew how to balance budgets, among other significant skills, people who knew how to "make things happen." Their primary activities in this facility were tea parties, crafts, bingo games or, the very worst, sitting by the window where they stared at nothing. I hated to see this waste of their life experience, wisdom, and willingness to return to the marketplace, as the Zen ox-herding tale describes, *with help-bestowing hands*, if not in active duty at least as consultants — wise elders.

I found and continue to find comfort that there are no signs that say "Need Not Apply" on the door marked "Sacred Activism" for those of us over 65. In fact, and as a proponent of the adage "Old age and treachery trumps youth and beauty," I believe that though any and all may engage in sacred activism, only the seasoned metal that has endured the most intense flame is destined to become the vehicle for healing and transformation so desperately required in our world today.

In addition, the sheer bulk of the numbers suggests that elders are a next vast "natural resource" to be tapped and utilized for great good. This demographic of elders around the globe is ripe and ready to undergo "the massive transformation in consciousness" to which Harvey calls us — a shift away from the limits of materialism in which we seem ensnared to a consciousness open to the infinity of Spirit. The down-to-earth words of Maggie Kuhn, founder of the Gray Panthers, point the way for those willing to become pioneers in this shift in consciousness:

> Older people are not just card-carrying members of Leisure World and mid-afternoon nap-takers. We are tribal elders, with an ongoing responsibility for safeguarding the tribe's survival and protecting the health of the planet. To do this, we must become society's futurists, testing out new instruments, technologies, ideas, and styles of living. We have the freedom to do so, and we have nothing to lose.

Harvey urges us to find our sacred passion. To do this, he warns us not to follow our bliss but, rather, *to follow our heartbreak*. What prevents us from doing this? Why do we find ourselves paralyzed, contracted with fear as we survey the rapidly escalating chaos before us?

In answer to the matter of fear, I suggest — and not glibly — that fear is a four-letter word like many others — good, hope, love, to name a few. A popular definition of "F.E.A.R." suggests this unpleasant emotion is nothing more than "false evidence appearing real." One of the great gifts of elderhood lies in the fact that we would not have arrived at this point in life had we not stood nose to nose with fear in about all of the forms it can take, not the least of which is that of death. Remember Maggie Kuhn: We've got nothing to lose and everything to gain as we step into our role as tribal elders, sacred activists.

Yes, the crises we face are many — the insanity of political discourse, the fragility of global economies, the collapse of institutional structures that dispense such "goods" as medicine, education, and law. In combination with staggering unemployment and environmental devastation, the choice of "Leisure World and afternoon naps" may well appear attractive. However, as Joe Lewis reminds us, we can run but we can't hide. Elder sacred activists understand that to hide in the face of global crisis is not an option. How many times have we heard the saying, "We're the ones we've been waiting for"?

The authentic spirituality to which Harvey is calling us demands a commitment to do something: to follow our heartbreak, not our bliss. If crisis and opportunity are two sides of the same coin, what is the one opportunity that masquerades as a crisis — the opportunity that breaks our hearts — here, now? Why stand on the sidelines, overwhelmed by the number and immensity of the challenges our culture faces? Identifying a commitment to one particular issue is unlikely to require that we think long or hard. In fact, each person who has achieved elder status has likely devoted considerable time, energy, and treasure to at least one source of heartbreak over the course of their lifetime, either through their professional or personal experience.

Wisdom gleaned in the trenches is invaluable, especially if elder sacred activists align their efforts as a global collective. Could this not spark the massive transformation in consciousness that Harvey is urging? Chaos theory tells us that any small, localized disturbance in one part of a complex system creates widespread effects throughout the whole system — the "butterfly effect." As I write these words, I wonder about the effect if, tomorrow morning, all over the globe, elders awoke to the power of their sacred activism and flapped their wings. What if each one of us engaged in one action followed by another and another to heal the issue that breaks our hearts? What magnitude of tsunami would such a wave of action create on behalf of the greater good?

While certainly tinted by the urgency Harvey voices, the vision I hold as an elder sacred activist reaches across time to embrace an inevitable infinity. The collective consciousness of our species has been evolving for a long time. Read the opening verses of the third book of *The Mahabharata*,[2] written in the 4th century BCE, and you will find its description of the chaos threatening to engulf the Earth eerily contemporary. Harvey's dire warning that our species is both out of time and out of grace is meant to prod us to action. However, against his dire prediction, I wish to suggest that the notion that "the end is near" works on one level only, that of the material world.

Not being much of a "Material Girl," my elder eyes see through the terrifying and chaotic illusion in the reality around me and find in the shape a deeper truth. "We are not human beings having a spiritual experience; we are spiritual beings having a human experience," Teilhard de Chardin observed. Thus, what does or doesn't happen to human inhabitants and the planet becomes irrelevant. The variable that does have eternal relevance here though, along with the invitation Andrew Harvey issued in his Pentecost workshop, is quite simply that of our dedication to live in service of Spirit.

What a Long, Strange Trip It's Been

by Edith Kusnic

OVER THE PAST FEW YEARS an image has been slowly forming in my mind, an image that paints a picture for me of the remarkable collective history of my generation's lifetime. One of the pleasantly surprising gifts of aging is this much broader perspective that allows one to see the Big Story of one's life and the times and their inextricable interconnection. It's as if pieces of a puzzle have slowly become visible one by one. With enough of them visible, it becomes possible to make out the whole picture.

This long view has much to offer us as we step into and through our elder years. Letting it inform our choices about how we spend the time that remains is increasingly urgent.

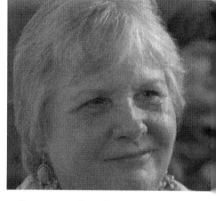

In 2009 I led an elders' retreat, Stepping into Elderhood, with a small group of folks, most of them in their early- or mid-sixties. After exploring our personal stories, we took a look at our common story by creating a visual timeline of our collective social history. All our concrete recollections — local, national, and international events; customs, fashion, music; every sort of thing — we posted on a big wall. Then we tried to make sense of it all. What was this era we had all lived through and that created the landscape within which our lives took place?

We realized we were the Atomic Generation, the first generation to grow up in the shadow of "The Bomb" (note the capitalization). Uncertain exactly how that fact impinged on our lives, we were nonetheless sure it had had incredible influences.

As we explored our shared social history, a clearer picture began to emerge. Our generation came of age during the tumultuous sixties, inspired and challenged by tectonic social changes: the Civil Rights struggle for human dignity; the quest for peace of the anti-war movement; and the dawning awareness, spurred by the environmental movement, of our connection with the more-than-human world.

As we moved into the seventies and eighties, we watched our youthful idealism be mocked and minimized. A new story of the sixties gained currency: We were a generation of hopeless, irrelevant idealists who didn't understand the real world and whose major concerns were sex, drugs, and rock and roll. And that was the positive spin!

The more negative view was that we were a failed generation who had not brought about the changes we dreamed of in the sixties — a world of peace and justice, a world where the promise of democracy would be realized for all people in this country and where solutions for the problems we faced would be found.

Looking now at the world of 2011, things do look like one big mess. In the late eighties, my young adult son said to me, "Don't talk to me about all your ideals and all that stuff. Your generation gave up. Things got hard and you just walked away." Clearly that's part of the prevailing myth. But is that really what happened? Did we just walk away? Or did we find places to put our energy and ways to begin to work toward the world we had imagined? Certainly, some did walk away, and others got lost along the way; but many of us sought ways to put our values into action.

What if we began to see and tell a different story of our life and times that challenges the prevailing story? Instead of seeing ourselves as a failed or inept generation, could we see ourselves as the forward wave in an immense tsunami of cultural change, a time of transition for human culture as it moves toward a new stage of development? When we look at our lives in this light, we may see the work of our generation as unfinished, gain energy and strength to continue our work with renewed vigor, and gain clarity about the work that is needed as we complete our lives' work.

What caught my imagination in the social history timeline we constructed in that 2009 elders' retreat was a picture of social and cultural forces flowing through our lives. I imagine a huge field of new energy coming into the world in the sixties; people everywhere inspired to imagine a wholly different form of human organization — a modern world, yes, but a world worthy of the dignity of human beings, a world that fosters the best of the human spirit. Cultural historian Thomas Berry characterized the "Great Work" of our times as nothing less than the reinventing of the human species. I think our generation in fact glimpsed this call to reinvent the human species.

As young people are wont to do, we set ourselves apart in dress and appearance. For many, however, this outward symbol marked a much deeper transformation, as many saw ourselves, albeit dimly, as the harbingers of a new reality.

Few people were immune from the energy unleashed during the sixties. The times were, indeed, "a-changin'" — as the civil rights movement, the war on poverty, the women's movement, the anti-war movement, the environmental movement, and many, many others began to transform our society. Change was also manifest in the music, in the "hippie" culture that was born, and in the burgeoning interest in Eastern religions. But the long register of positive developments was also balanced by negative ones: violence, drug abuse, the collapse of faith in social and political institutions, a divided country.

As the seventies gave way to the eighties, the backlash of reaction coalesced into a strong political force of its own. Those advocating the "new way" became increasingly marginalized. On the surface of the culture, hair got cut, suits put on, and the childish things of the sixties were put away. Reagan became president, and order was restored.

But ferment continued beneath the surface. The unleashed energy had brought intimations of what is possible in the human realm along with vague directions and clues about how to pursue it. Like a vision that comes to one fasting in the wilderness, it needed much interpretation and a lot of time to understand it. If we challenge the cynical story of our generation, perhaps we can see that the field of energy let loose in the sixties was not extinguished or burned out. It went underground, carried by those of us who had experienced it.

In this picture we see ourselves as having lived through a cultural rite of passage — born into and living through this time of immense cultural change that was the second half of the twentieth century. For us, the old world passed away as we were moving along the path to adulthood. But the new world was yet to be born. We have found ourselves, throughout our lives, as standing between two worlds, always living with the question of what kind of new world will emerge.

Eco-philosopher and teacher Joanna Macy identifies three streams of work necessary for shifting our culture to a life-sustaining one. First are holding actions, the work needed to blunt destructive practices and policies and mitigate the suffering they cause. Dealing with the consequences of homelessness, opposing wars, and advocating sane actions against climate change are examples of this stream. The second challenge is building new forms, the work of creating new social forms and practices and developing the conceptual understanding necessary for them. Examples of this have been the alternative health movement, the local and organic food movement, and work on alternative energy. The third stream Macy calls shifting consciousness and includes work in psychology, consciousness studies, and new spiritual and religious ideas and practices.

My daughter once characterized the people she knew from my generation as pathfinders who forged trails through new territory so that her generation could find its way more easily. Perhaps we should all see our generation this way. We didn't give up; rather we dispersed and began laying trails through these three streams of knowledge and action that Macy described. Some have worked to save habitat and wilderness areas, others have taken on poverty and economic injustice, war, or toxins in the environment. Still others have focused on alternative energy, new forms of education, or building new structures for cooperative living. Other folks have explored new spiritual understandings and worked to build a bridge between the secular and spiritual. And that is just the beginning. When we begin to look more closely, we can see evidence of people who have been hard at work for years laying a foundation for a new way of thinking needed to meet the challenges of the future. Often, however, this has taken place below the radar of mainstream media and attention.

But at the same time we can also see the evidence of the strength of the forces that have vehemently opposed the kind of change we sought. Social, environmental, and political problems we began to identify in the sixties have festered and grown more virulent. Our political system is broken, our economy in tatters, the effects of global climate change already in evidence. In short, we all know that we have made a grand mess of things and, even if we have different interpretations of what and why and how, we all know that something is terribly wrong.

As I write this in the late fall of 2011, news of the Occupy movement is finally being covered on mainstream news. Like many other demonstrations and protests that since the seventies have been tagged as originating from the "Left," it was ignored for many weeks by the mainstream press and disparaged and denigrated by those on the Right. In the revived epithets we hear clear echoes of the sixties: "Dirty Hippies!" "Get a job!" "Take a bath." "Anti-American!" "Socialists!" "Communist!" It's been over 40 years since the height of that era's "young people's uprising," but those anachronistic slogans are once again marshaled to keep us locked into a fraudulent story of our generation. Meanwhile, it is business as usual toward planetary destruction.

Most recently the coverage of the Occupy movement has been about the over-the-top police response and what appears to be a concerted effort nationwide to stop the movement. As I watched the video of the pepper spray incident in Davis, California, I flashed back to the image of the young girl at Kent State bent over the body of a young man, one of four shot dead by National Guardsmen, and remembered the shooting of students two weeks later at Jackson State (two dead and twelve injured). Iconic images of college students — our nation's young people — bearing the brunt of military-style policing 41 years apart. The shadow of the sixties is visible across the country. The forces amassed to repress this latest attempt to visibly bring forth new values are strong.

But the Occupy movement also brings a new glimmer of hope. Is this the moment we have been waiting for all our lives? The moment when consciousness shifts, a new Zeitgeist appears, and suddenly we are united in working for a better future for all of us? Can this become that moment — not the moment of a grand ideological struggle where the battles of the sixties continue to be fought, but the moment when we move beyond them, together finding new solutions to entrenched problems? Or will we continue on the old path, allowing problems to continue to fester, leaving challenges unmet? What a heroic struggle is taking place in our body politic, not between Right and Left, but between hope and cynicism!

I don't want to inflate our importance, but I think that answering these questions may be the unfinished work of our generation and the key to choosing between the two paths open to us. I also think that in finishing that work we will be completing our generation's story, finally stepping fully into our responsibility for our culture and our world. Many of us were denied that completion as we stepped into adulthood. The gifts we brought were disdained by a mainstream culture desperately opposed to change. But if we are strategic and conscious, our elder years may offer the opportunity to complete our work.

A few years ago I encountered the "Awakening the Dreamer, Changing the Dream" symposium designed by The Pachamama Alliance. The ambitious mission of that symposium is "To bring forth an environmentally sustainable, spiritually fulfilling, and socially just human presence on the planet." What struck me most were the words "to bring forth." I realized that bringing forth requires an orientation that has often been missing for many of us in our generation. We have often been held in the position of children, dismissed and disdained, mocked and minimized as naïve idealists. As we tried to bring forth the values and knowledge that came into our consciousness in the sixties, we were met with riot police and eventually guns. As a generation, we were not welcomed by our elders and encouraged to bring our gifts into the larger community. We were told to be quiet and fit in, if we wanted a place in the community of adults.

The similarities between the Occupy movement and the movements of the sixties are striking, but there are also key differences. An important difference is that this current generation of young people — those sleeping in tents across the country, suffering abuse, and getting arrested — have elders who share their values. We can welcome them into adulthood, valuing what they have to offer. We can mentor them; we can offer to share the skills and knowledge gathered on our own underground journeys. In short, we can be the elders all of us needed and few of us got.

Another difference is that the slogans thrown around this time no longer seem to have the power they once had. They're beginning to ring hollow. More and more people trust the evidence of their own eyes and ears. Schoolteachers and cops and firemen are not Communists bent on overthrowing the government. They are not wastrels, living on the dole.

But the forces that want us to adopt the other story are strong and very well organized. For over 40 years they have been effective at characterizing — as somehow a left-wing Communist plot — the basic human work of living up to one's values, trying to make the world a better place, and living in harmony and balance with the wider natural world.

Perhaps, in our elder years, we can change the orientation we adopted and cease to see ourselves as simply advocates for the world we imagined all those years ago. Instead, we are those with the knowledge and skills needed for building that world.

Perhaps by stepping fully into our roles as elders we can help shift the tide and allow a New Story to be written. Perhaps by naming and claiming the story of our own generation, we will be telling the stories the young ones need to hear. Perhaps by naming and claiming what we've learned during these past 40 years we will be passing it on to a new generation actively trying to overcome the cynicism and gridlock that holds this country in its grip.

We've learned in many ways and in many different arenas what it means to be a human being and the conditions necessary for humans to thrive and reach their full potential. We've learned about how to communicate, cooperate, and collaborate to create social forms that nurture the human spirit. We've glimpsed spiritual understandings that unite instead of divide. We've learned about what hurts our precious planet Earth and what nurtures it and us. We've learned so much in our individual journeys as pathfinders — so much which will help create an "environmentally sustainable, spiritually fulfilling, and socially just human presence on the planet."

Now appears the time to find ways to share what we've learned and nurture a new generation struggling to find hope and the will to action — struggling to find a way to transcend the cynicism and despair rampant in our times. To do that, we must step fully into conscious, intentional elderhood, taking responsibility for the future. This may well be the path of redemption and fulfillment for our generation — the action needed to finish our generation's work and help put this nation on the track that will lead to the world we have been imagining all our lives.

The *Bhagavad Gita* has been a constant companion since I first began studying it over 20 years ago. Considered a core yogic text, the Gita speaks directly to suffering and liberation. It is a manual of spiritual instruction, an allegory for the struggle between higher and lower instincts, and a cautionary tale on the consequences of not following one's dharma or true path. Both Gandhi and Henry David Thoreau found the Gita to be indispensable. I began with the translation by Eknath Easwaran (Nilgiri Press), which I still love, but Stephen Mitchell's more recent version (Three Rivers Press) is pure poetry. From chapter 9:

I am the beginning and the end,
origin and dissolution,
refuge, home, true lover,
womb and imperishable seed.

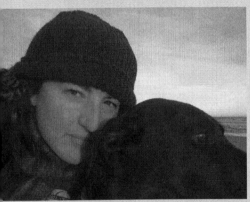

Claudia Horwitz and Zak

Claudia Horwitz founded **stone circles** at The Stone House in 1995 to strengthen and sustain people working for transformation and justice. The Stone House is one of the first land-based centers in the country uniting spiritual practice, social justice, and land stewardship. After 17 years as Executive Director, she now serves as a teacher, trainer, writer, speaker, and weaver of work focused on spiritual activism. She is the author of *The Spiritual Activist: Practices to Transform Your Life, Your Work, and Your World* (Penguin Compass, 2002).

How Can YOU Help?

by Robert C. Atchley

FOR MANY PEOPLE, SERVICE — voluntarily giving aid or comfort to others — is a spiritual experience. The motive and action of service connects them with their deeper, transpersonal spiritual nature. The capacity to perceive the spiritual aspects of everyday experience develops throughout life and usually reaches its highest levels in later life. So it is no surprise that the spiritual side of service assumes more importance as people age.

Much attention has been given to the assertion that aging baby boomers constitute an enormous reserve of experienced people who might have a profound effect on the quality of humanitarian work being done in our communities. My thesis is that such service is primarily motivated by the fact that for many people *service is a spiritual experience*. There is a fundamental link between spiritual development (a growing capacity to perceive the spiritual elements of experience), years of life experience that has been well reflected upon, and capacity for spiritually centered community service.

In their book, *How Can I Help?*, Ram Dass and Paul Gorman (1985) assert that service stems from the human impulse to care. We can see this especially clearly in how communities respond to disasters such as floods or tornadoes. At such times, the impulse to care for one another is overwhelming. The impulse to care is a noble inclination, but it tells us little about how to care or what will be effective. Service over the long run requires that we build on the impulse to care.

A model of spiritually enlightened service begins with the need to be spiritually grounded as we serve. This means that each of us must attend to our inner spirituality. The spiritual journey involves finding and exploring our particular spiritual path and seeking experiences that open us to the vastness of inner space. As we grow spiritually, we develop levels of consciousness and awareness that alert us to the obstacles thrown in our path by self-centeredness. Ego-based service is first and foremost about the ego's needs. Enlightened service rises above the ego to more clearly see what is needed. Moving toward enlightened service requires developing the skill needed to remain spiritually centered as we go about our work.

Many well-intentioned people find their service less satisfying than they would like it to be because they do not have essential information about the structure and operation of the field in which they wish to serve. Most areas of service have their own unique concepts and language about what they do and how they do it. "Paying your dues" involves getting the experience needed to ensure being sufficiently informed to serve effectively. This does not mean passively accepting other people's definitions of what is good, true, or beautiful; it means thoroughly understanding the situation before weighing in with suggestions for change.

A person who is accomplished at serving from spirit is able to stay spiritually centered amid the ups and downs of working in an organizational environment, often in situations involving people who are in desperate need. It is essential to be very knowledgeable about how to work within the organizational context and with the types of people who are to be served.

Listen to Your Entire Being

People find their way to spiritual paths and to community service in a large variety of ways. The mind, the ego, the heart, the body, and the soul can each lead us. But if we are only listening to one part of being, then we are not taking advantage of all our resources for being clear about what we are doing, or thinking about doing. Listening to your entire being means cultivating sensitivity to each dimension of being. This possibility is greatly enhanced by contemplative practice — meditation, rumination, and inner stillness and quietude. In this sense, contemplative practice is an important companion on both the inner spiritual journey and the outer journey of service. Contemplative practice can put us in touch with higher levels of consciousness, from which it is possible to see clearly the workings of the mind and the ego, our true compassion, actions that would truly be of service, and a pace that is healthy for the body.

Mindfulness and Transcendence

Mindfulness and transcendence are important qualities to bring to the spiritual journey and to bring to service. *Mindfulness* is being right here, right now. It is an intense awareness of the present moment. With mindfulness we are able to see more clearly what is before us. We are more likely to see what will actually be helpful in serving another human being or serving an organization. In this framework, it is not so much a matter of doing for others as *you* would like to be done for, but doing for others as *they* would like. It is a matter of doing service that is not self-centered.

To employ mindful service, we also need a vantage point that transcends our ordinary consciousness of self. Ordinary consciousness is ego-centered. We are the main character in the drama. But as soon as we begin to *witness* our ordinary self, we have transcended that self and can see it more clearly than we possibly could from the middle of our ego-agendas of desire or fear. To the witness, we are only one of the characters in the drama and not necessarily the most important one at a given moment.

Becoming Wisdom and Compassion in Action

BEING WISE AND HAVING COMPASSION are not all-or-nothing. They are *qualities* that exist in degrees. They are not something we have, they are *capacities* we can develop. They are qualities that we *might* be able to bring into being to a given situation. If we have cultivated wisdom and compassion, then we have a greater capacity to manifest those qualities, but this happens in the present moment. Whether we can manifest wisdom and compassion depends on how centered we can remain. When we are in a situation of service, we are usually called to be wise and to be compassionate. How well we can do this depends a great deal on how long we have been practicing wisdom and compassion.

Often we think of service as something that involves volunteering or working within an organizational context. However, service is really an intention that we can take with us into a wide variety of situations we find ourselves in. What would happen if we went joyfully about our daily lives seeing every person as someone we could potentially serve, in however small a way? What would happen if we took every opportunity to tend our planet and our environment? Many times these are not big programs or long-term tasks but instead are things we can do moment, by moment, by moment. It only takes a few minutes to deeply listen to someone who needs a receptive ear; it only takes a few seconds to pick up a piece of trash. The feeling of service is something that happens in the present moment, whether you are doing it in an organizational context or purely on your own.

Paying Dues

EACH NEW SERVICE ENVIRONMENT we enter has its own language and customs, and we need to give ourselves time to assimilate these elements. Otherwise we risk behaving in ways that seem arrogant, naïve, or clueless to those already working in the environment. Curiosity and humility provide a useful stance from which to pay one's dues and earn the respect of others in the environment. Be careful about assuming that knowledge from another field can be readily adapted to a new situation. Ask lots of questions and ask for help learning the ropes.

Much of our service occurs in an organizational context. What are the mission and vision of the organization? What values serve to anchor the operation of the organization? What are the major goals of the organization? What outcomes does the organization seek? To what extent are the clients involved in setting goals? Who are the major stakeholders in the success of the organization? These and many other questions create a big picture within which your work will take place. It's important to know how your work fits into the whole.

Take Care of Yourself

Effective service is based in a balance between caring for others and caring for oneself. We all need rest, nourishment, and perspective if we are to be able to serve over the long run. Rest is not just sleep, although sleep is very important. Rest also occurs when we pace ourselves so we are not living in a perpetually rushed state. Nourishment of the body is equally important, but so is nourishment of the mind and spirit. Contemplative reading of sacred texts or books and articles on spiritual themes is an example of a practice that nourishes the mind. Meditation is an example of a restful practice that nourishes the spirit. Leading a contemplative life aimed at nurturing the whole person provides a perspective that allows us to bring enough love to our acts of service that we can endure the pain of compassion.

Does Life Stage Matter?

IF WE THINK ABOUT STAGES of adulthood in terms of issues and challenges of young adulthood, middle age, later adulthood, and old age, then there are major differences in (1) competition from interests other than community service, (2) effects of the amount and type of life experience, and (3) interest in an intentional spiritual journey.

In young adulthood, people often focus on finding a livelihood that is right for them and making decisions about mate selection and family formation. By the time people reach middle age, their job and family responsibilities often become routine, perhaps still demanding but well within their capacity, and opportunities for community involvement often increase. In later adulthood, having launched children into adulthood and having retired from the workforce can bring increased freedom to choose a life of community service. In old age, many people maintain their involvement in community organizations, especially religious organizations, and some find themselves serving as sages and spiritual elders.

In terms of the interPart of spirituality and community service, young adults often experience strong pressures to concentrate on employment and family, both of which can mobilize the impulse to care. For many young adults, issues concerning the meaning of life have not yet stimulated them to think about a conscious spiritual journey. By the end of young adulthood, most people have had enough experience living with the results of their own actions to have deep respect for the difficulties of deciding a right course of action.

By middle age, many adults have begun to question our materialistic culture's definitions of the good life. Many have followed society's prescription for life satisfaction only to find the results less than satisfying. They may then embark on a search for meaning, and the world's wisdom traditions offer many spiritual paths for finding it. At the same time, increased opportunities for community involvement and service can provide an experience of meaning through service. The spiritual journey and the journey of service usually complement one another.

Later adulthood can also bring a need for new direction. Those who did not develop an orientation to serving from spirit in midlife may find themselves drawn to it later, as child launching and retirement create opportunities to rethink one's lifestyle. After a period of resting up from the demands of middle age, many people at the beginning of later adulthood begin a period of experimenting with various ways to lead a satisfying life. Eventually, some settle into a life focused around community service.

In old age, there are adults who are uniquely qualified to serve as sages and/or spiritual elders — individuals who combine a deep spiritual connection, insights based in their considerable life experience, and concern for nurturing the upcoming generations of adults. As parents, many spiritual elders help ease the transition of their offspring into later adulthood. They serve as role models and mentors for middle-aged and older adults as well as for young people. Spiritual elders continue to participate in the life of the community, but they often have moved beyond the need to take an operational leadership role.

Bon Voyage

I'VE COVERED A LOT OF GROUND in this essay, but I hope it gives you food for thought as you think about your own journey of spiritual development and how it ties into your impulse to care for others and our planet. If you want further reading on spiritually grounded service, *How Can I Help?*, by Ram Dass and Paul Gorman (Alfred A. Knopf, 1995), is an excellent place to start.

Healing the World

by Judith Helburn

I came to introspection late in life. The whirlwind of life was too exciting, too invigorating for me to slow down enough to look within. For me, it was about action. I was a doer. I didn't know that to be a whole being, I also needed stillness and quiet. I didn't know that I needed to listen to inner voices as well as those out there. Yet, through the first seasons of my years, I was seeking I knew not what. It was in the autumn of my life — in what my teacher and mentor, Rabbi Zalman Schachter-Shalomi, calls "harvest time" — that I realized that one could both do and be. I discovered the Kabbalah and the story of the shards of Divine Light which gave me focus. The story explained my own desire to balance doing and being.

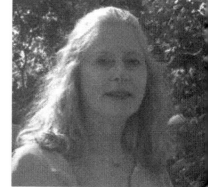

Isaac Luria, a sixteenth-century Kabbalist, used the phrase "Tikkun Olam" (which is usually translated as "repairing the world") to encapsulate the true role of humanity in the ongoing evolution and spiritualization of the cosmos. Luria taught that God created the world and formed vessels to hold the Divine Light with which to finalize the work. But as God poured Light into the vessels, they shattered, tumbling down and carrying Light sparks toward our newly formed world. By doing good deeds and helping to mend the world, we are able to discover the shards and the sparks and grow closer to that which is holy.

> "…[O]ur personal inner work makes a difference. If we can raise ourselves to the station where the Divine can see and act through us, then we complete the momentous work of restoring at least one part to the Whole.…"[1]

Based on the premise that by healing ourselves, we heal the world and vice versa, what is the next step? First, we are only expected to do our part.

> It is not incumbent on thee to finish the work,
> but neither art thou permitted to desist from it altogether.
> — *Pirkei Avot*

Where do we begin? I'm not certain that it matters. However, if we are content and happy, we are more likely to reach out to others. According to a study by the British Office for National Statistics, happiness is made up of knowing oneself and contributing to society. Other studies show that helping others helps us to live longer. Helping others moves us beyond ego, puts our own lives in perspective. Positive attitudes help our immune systems. Sharing our stories with other generations connects us to the future. Our stories help others to find precedents for dealing with the Unknown. It is one way of giving back.

David Brooks states in an interview by Charlie Rose about his recent book, *The Social Animal*, that we have a desire to merge with the other, be it another person or even God. There is happiness in connecting. He elaborated further in an Op Ed column in *The New York Times* (March 2011):

> We are social animals, deeply interpenetrated with one another, who emerge out of relationships.... [Our] unconscious mind hungers for those moments of transcendence when the skull line falls away and we are lost in love for another, the challenge of a task or the love of God.

Grace is what happens when we let go of our egos and open ourselves. In the "harvest time" of later life, we have access to wisdom from the heart, not just the head. The demands of daily life ease a bit, and we as elders have more time to do our inner work. Even when what we work towards doesn't happen, something else does, opening up new possibilities.

Martin Luther King put it this way: "An individual has not started living until he can rise above the narrow confines of his individualistic concerns to the broader concerns of all humanity."

Reb Zalman put it this way: "If my outer world is degraded, then my inner world is degraded." The moral imperative for me is that I must reach out. I must give back. Eric Erikson believed that Generativity,[2] the act of contributing to society and helping to guide future generations, was the single most important function of old age.

I do so by helping people be the best they can be in the second half of life. I lead a monthly "learn and lunch" for the Second Sixty of my Jewish community. I have facilitated a women's memoir writing circle for 14 years. I introduce Sage-ing or vital aging anywhere and everywhere I can. More importantly, I try to live Sage-ing as who I am.

One can be of service even unconsciously. I have volunteered to work (and play) in an Alzheimer's Respite Care group meeting once a week. Of course, that is a service needed and appreciated, but what a great gift it has given me! I have discovered that my unacknowledged fear of dementia has diminished considerably. The people with whom I work are, for the most part, charming, fun, and able to carry on interesting conversations. It is their memories which they are losing at this point, not their personalities and their intelligence. They are not conscious of their gift to me, but I am. I have learned to listen. Sarah Lawrence-Lightfoot, a Harvard professor, recounts this lesson learned from Mary Catherine Bateson: "You must listen to your daughter — she is from another planet, and she has a great deal to teach you." We must not only listen. We must continue to learn from others, old and young.

I am concerned for our planet. I do what I can — recycling, conserving energy, creating a small haven for animals and birds in my own yard, living mindfully. As I have aged, I have found that my needs and desires have lessened. I look beyond what it is that I want to what is best for the greater community. I have a cartoon from Sally Forth in which the family is planting a tree. Sally explains to a neighborhood child that the tree will bear fruit in the future — for others.

The buzz of my earlier life is no more. My energy and enthusiasm continue, but I am a quieter presence now. Making a difference makes me feel good. And when I feel good, I feel connected to all that is.

Getting There

It took over half a century for my selves
to fit comfortably inside this familiar skin

The Curious Child
questioned everything

The Mute Poet sang freely
undaunted by mirrors

The Everlasting Learner
learned how much she had to teach

The Clown dropped her crutches
to join freely in the dance

The Fool found the wisdom
to become her own best friend

The Storyteller spun tales
part myths, part truths

The Parent abdicated their futures
to her daughters and her sons

The Evangelist laughed
abandoning the crusades

The Advocate
stopped playing god

The Pacifist fought
to find inner peace

And the old Survivor
healed her wounds with words
    — Lorna Louise Bell[†]

[†] Published in *Celebrating Poets over 70*, M. Vespry and E. Ryan, editors (McMaster Centre for Gerontological Studies, 2010).

Jock Brandis:
Championing Stone Age Technology
by Pat and Steve Taylor

> *In the face of a possible nuclear holocaust and the rape of the earth and the obscene poverty of whole peoples... it is time to reconsider what life is really all about.*
> — Joan Chittister

JOOST (JOCK) BRENDER A BRANDIS, a Dutch native who grew up in Canada and now resides in Wilmington, North Carolina, has created a Universal Nut Sheller, a device called "the holy grail of sustainable agriculture." With this invention, and the several others that followed, he is considered one of the world's leading authorities in the emerging field of appropriate technology.

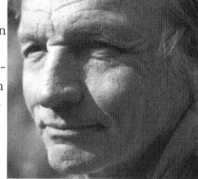

Jock has been interested in technological innovation since his undergraduate service as a cadet in the Canadian Naval ROTC. That fascination continued in his first career as an electrical technician and lighting director for dozens of major motion pictures. One of his oft-repeated stories involves his on-the-set creation of a carnivorous bed from air mattresses, food coloring, and Mr. Bubble foam. His encore career — to which he promises to devote as much time and energy as he did to his work on movie crews — began after the death of his wife from cancer in 1995 and his decision to remain close to home to care for his young children, then 9 and 14.

When asked by a friend for advice in fashioning a solar-powered irrigation system for a village in Mali, he gathered various components and flew to Africa to oversee the installation.

While there, he noticed that the women of the village had bloody fingers from hours spent shelling their main cash crop, peanuts. He promised that he would send them an inexpensive peanut sheller, but when he returned home, he discovered that everything on the market required some sort of electrical power source. The nearest electric service was many miles away from these village women, so Jock invented a device that can be operated by simply turning a crank on the top.

To most Americans, shelling a peanut may seem neither difficult nor meaningful, but in Sub-Saharan Africa, some half a billion people in dozens of countries depend on the peanut as a primary source of protein, livelihood, soil restoration, and rural economies. And the variety of peanut that grows there is so difficult to remove from its shell that the women who spend half of their lives at such labor become progressively crippled.

His creation, which he modestly refers to as "Stone Age technology," uses $28 worth of materials and can be manufactured on site from a kit assembled by volunteers in his Wilmington, North Carolina, workshop. He quickly interested a group of Peace Corps veterans in forming a nonprofit called Full Belly Project which would distribute the shellers. Meanwhile, he was tweaking the invention so that it would operate not only on peanuts, but also on coffee beans, pistachios, and, perhaps most significantly, jatropha seeds, which can now be used to produce diesel fuel, fertilizer, and a natural insecticide.

As Jock realized the tremendous effect his invention had on people's lives, he moved on to other simple and inexpensive machines. His gentle manner, old-world charm, and humility won over philanthropic people from many countries and allowed him to attract volunteers and grant money to Full Belly Project. He also has earned the trust of native peoples around the world whom he has trained in the manufacture and operation of his machines. They have become social entrepreneurs and manufacturers in 17 countries.

Mali, Haiti, and the Philippines are among the beneficiaries of his ingenuity, but not the only ones. His latest device was invented to solve a problem he found closer to home. In Rutherford County, North Carolina, small farmers needed a simple way to get water to their farms for irrigation and livestock consumption. These farms are bordered by small creeks — themselves tributaries of larger rivers that feed reservoirs of the larger cities in Central North and South Carolina. The streams, however, are fenced, both to control erosion and to prevent the livestock from fouling the water. To solve the farmers' problem, Jock ran pipe beneath the fencing and created a gravity-powered water pump to siphon the water from the stream. Again, he used only readily available materials: PVC pipe and rubber gaskets made from used truck tire inner tubes.

The sandy-haired, greying 6-footer with blue eyes that twinkle when he talks about his projects likes to work quickly. He admits that he hears "time's winged chariot," and he feels he has much left to do in adapting wind, solar, water, and human power to the problems of the developing world. He also recognized early on the importance of replicability, and so he has created what he calls the "factory in a box." He and his volunteers ship the designs and instructions for assembly, along with the basic components, to dozens of villages each month to make problem-solving entrepreneurs of the local people.

Allen Armstrong, an engineering professor at M.I.T., notes that Jock's Universal Nut Sheller is entirely new — new shape, new materials, and a new method of manufacturing. Moreover, his work is beginning to change the way international development is done — away from large corporate centers often far removed from its beneficiaries, and toward smaller, local groups with simple products. These simpler devices use low-cost, locally available materials, and can be operated and maintained with a minimum of training by local people. Jock is currently working with the National Geographic Society and a Philippines philanthropist to come up with a school building that can be made from plastic bottles.

Jock is one of those people who has thought deeply about the purpose of life, so deeply and yet so emotionally that, in 2008, he was the recipient of a $100,000 cash award. Bestowed annually to those who are "taking matters into their own hands and fashioning a new vision of the second half of life," the Purpose Prize arrived just in time for him to keep his home from foreclosure. For most of his life, he has possessed few material goods. In our family, he is often called a modern St. Francis, because, like Francis of Assisi, he trusts that the universe will provide. Once, when he was several months in arrears on his house payment and was literally days from foreclosure, an unknown woman appeared at his door, told him she had seen a Canadian Broadcasting Corporation video about his work, and handed him a check that more than covered his delinquent payments.

Jock is the quintessential optimist, which helps him develop new ideas. Studies have shown that hopefulness and optimism lengthen life. Those who are dynamically engaged, full of plans, working toward meaningful accomplishment are almost guaranteed a longer life span. Jock is also a good listener. Each day, in his workshop, he is surrounded by volunteers, from high school students to senior citizens, eager to learn practical things — how to weld steel, mix concrete, and assemble PVC — but also to expose their ideas to Jock's problem-solving analysis and technological know-how.

His work has touched the lives of a diverse group of people, from African village elders using machines adapted from old bicycles, to Indian farmers using foot-powered water pumps, to M.I.T. graduate students eager to learn how to think outside the box, to former President Jimmy Carter (a man who knows a thing or two about peanuts himself). Several short documentary films have been produced about his work.

He has inspired many to imitate him. Ming Leong, an M.I.T. engineer who spent a summer as a Full Belly Project intern, says, "Just being around Jock has made me feel like, yeah, I have a chance to make a difference too."

Invitations to Practice

THE INNER WORK OF NONVIOLENCE
by Betsy Crites

> *Compassion and love are not mere luxuries. As the source both of inner and external peace, they are fundamental to the continued survival of our species.*
>
> — The Dalai Lama

Nonviolence as a means of societal transformation can be far more effective when the practitioners have also undertaken a discipline of personal transformation. By attending to our own mental and emotional states, such as anger, hatred, and aggression, and by working to create peaceful realms in our immediate circles, we simultaneously contribute to a world that supports nonviolence.

Nonviolence scholar, Michael Nagler notes that "Nonviolence begins in inner struggle — specifically, the struggle to keep anger, fear, and greed from having sway over us."[1] And Dr. King reminds us: "Nonviolence means avoiding not only external physical violence, but also internal violence of spirit. You not only refuse to shoot a man, but you refuse to hate him."[2]

To follow this maxim requires cultivating a spiritual discipline, which ideally includes regular time for reflection and meditation. Reflection on the wisdom of great spiritual leaders who aligned their actions with their high ideals expands our sense of what is possible. Meditation and prayer take us to that place of refuge where we can deepen our insight and strengthen our resolve.

A personal discipline of self-reflection can help us overcome the conditioning that keeps us thinking inside the box and acting reflexively. We are all subject to strong biases from within our culture and modern society. We are taught to think in terms of "we" against "them," and put our faith in zero-sum contests where the winner takes all. This model permeates our political, economic, and criminal justice systems.

Since we are shown violence at every turn — on TV and in movies, books, or other media — we tend to accept it as the norm. This is a misperception Gandhi frequently addressed:

> The fact that there are so many men still alive in the world shows that it is based not on force of arms but on the force of truth or love… Little quarrels of millions of families in their daily lives disappear before the exercise of this force. Hundreds of nations live in peace. History does not and cannot take note of this fact. History is really a record of the interruption of the even working of the force of love.[3]

Gandhi was trained as a lawyer. Through his painful experiences of discrimination in South Africa and his profound introspection and reflection, he managed to decondition himself from the elements of this training that picks winners against losers. He wrote about his "experiments in truth," which were in essence a long process of retraining himself and discovering the principles of nonviolence. It was not about learning the wisdom of others or acquiring intellectual understanding, though he certainly did that as well. What really shifted him and empowered him was the wisdom that arose out of his experience. S.N. Goenka, a Buddhist teacher from India, describes this as "the wisdom that one lives, real wisdom that will bring about a change in one's life by changing the very nature of the mind."[4]

When we peek outside the box of our competitive, violence-prone society, we might discover what Gandhi called, "the most powerful force the world has known," nonviolence.

Part IV

Rites of Passage into Elderhood

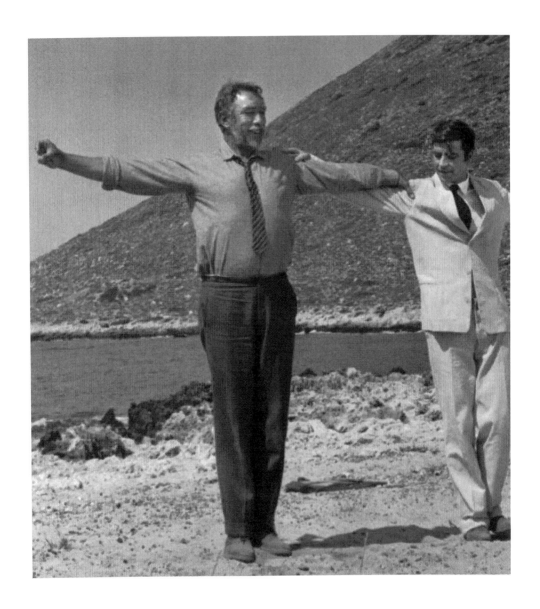

THE DANCE OF SPIRIT IN LATER LIFE

BY BOLTON ANTHONY

The task of life's first journey is to *construct* a competent ego that allows us to survive and succeed in the world: to find work — ideally, work that speaks to our deep passion and contributes to the greater good; to build mutually sustaining relationships with others and open ourselves to intimacy; and to nurture those in our care. The task of life's *second journey* is to *deconstruct* the ego we have assembled with such care or — perhaps, more accurately — to *slough it off*. This sort of *letting go* is possible, because the ego is merely the creation of the mind; it "has no existence by itself," as D.H. Lawrence writes, "It is only the glitter of the sun on the surface of the waters."[1]

Vision quest guide Bill Plotkin has called the first task our *survival dance*; and the second, our *sacred dance*.[2] Though we, of course, begin constructing our ego in earliest childhood, only at that first great transition point in life — when we move from adolescence to adulthood or, in the four Hindu stages of life, from Student to Householder — are we truly ready to learn our survival dance. *When the student is ready, the dance instructor will appear*. In traditional societies, the elders of the tribe always served as guides and teachers for this rite of passage that launches our first journey.

There is, of course, a second great transition point in life — when we are moving from midlife into elderhood (or from Householder to Forest Dweller). Now we are again ready to learn a new dance, our sacred dance. Here too, elders, in the guise of Sage, have served as guides for this rite of passage that launches our second journey.

Here are two famous literary examples of guides for this rite of passage:

> Virgil appears in the first canto of *The Inferno* to guide Dante, a midlife pilgrim who has wandered into "dark woods, the right road lost." Like most entering therapy, he wants help *now*! "See this beast driving me backward — help me *resist*," he begs.[3] But, again, the second journey is never about resistance — it's always about letting go, sloughing off. And because "the way up is the way down"[4] (more about this later), the path Virgil and Dante follow must first *descend* into hell.

It was in this same borderland — after another descent — that Odysseus, the long-suffering hero of Homer's *Odyssey*, encounters his guide, the blind seer Tiresias. After accurately prophesying the many trials and years of wandering that will precede Odysseus' return home, Tiresias lets him in on a secret: *there's more*. The encounter with Tiresias occurs in Book 11 of the *Odyssey's* 24 books; Odysseus remembers and recounts the seer's prophesy to his wife Penelope in Book 23. At this point in the epic, he has come home to Ithaca, driven the suitors out, and been reunited with his wife, son, and father. This is the "happy ever after" ending of his first journey. The secret Tiresias shares is that a second, different journey awaits Odysseus at the end of his life.[5]

So, there is this pattern: the *survival dance*, then the *sacred dance*. Learning our survival dance is the task of our first journey in life; learning our sacred dance, of our second. You cannot begin the second task — or, to use mystical language, you cannot *enter the kingdom of heaven*[6] — until you have done the first.

But there is also this paradox: Though our survival dance is about constructing an ego that allows us to "succeed in the world," if we wish to "graduate" and move on to our sacred dance, *we almost always need to fail at the task*.

That's because, as Richard Rohr writes, "*The way up is the way down. Or, if you prefer, the way down is the way up.*"[7] There is a story, perhaps apocryphal, about a patient that Carl Jung had been treating who would invariably show up for his sessions in the best of moods, everything going well, no complaints. This continued for some time, with the patient — in Jung's eyes — making only minimal progress. Then, finally, one day he shows up not doing well at all, a disastrous week, the world falling apart around him. Ah, Jung says to himself, *Now* we can get something done!

The film *Zorba the Greek* (1964) provides another wonderfully apt illustration. Basil, a young writer of Greek/English descent, arrives in Crete, having recently inherited a small cottage and a long-defunct lignite mine. Zorba — the figure of the sage guide in the film — attaches himself to the younger man, impressing him with his repertoire of indispensable skills, which he points out includes considerable mining expertise.

The Englishman is, of course, *stuck* — lost in midlife's "dark woods." His writer's block, which he hopes the solitude of Crete will help him break, is the symbol of a much larger emotional paralysis. A series of unmitigated disasters follow — all of them building to this final cathartic scene:

Zorba has constructed a cable line to transport timbers, logged from the stand of trees on the mountain above, down to the entrance to the mineshaft; these will be used to replace the rotting timbers which support timbers in the mine. The whole village gathers, including the abbot and priests from the nearby monastery who provide the necessary rituals of blessing. At Zorba's signal, the men at the top launch the first log, which gains speed as it travels down and breaks apart. But since it does make it to where Zorba stands at the head of the mine, he tells Basil, "Don't worry," and fires the rifle a second time. A second, larger log careens down the singing cable. People scramble out of the way, some of them diving into the sea where the log finally lands. Again (though with tempered bravado) Zorba reassures Basil, "It's nothing," and fires the rifle again. With the onslaught of this last log, each brace in turn gives way; everyone scatters, and the entire structure collapses in a dusty explosion.

Here is a litany of what has happened to Basil: The widow who invited him to her bed has died, stoned to death by the jealous villagers; his patrimony, the mine, has proved worthless; his small inheritance has been used up. All has collapsed in a magnificent, "splendiferous crash." (*Now we can get something done!*) It is only at this moment — only when everything lies in shambles — that Basil can say to Zorba: "Teach me to dance" — not my survival dance, my sacred dance.

Let us turn now to two stories of initiation — a short story, "The Artificial Nigger," by the Southern writer Flannery O'Connor, and the 2003 French film, *Monsieur Ibrahim*. Both, on the surface at least, involve the rite of passage of an adolescent into adulthood. Let us explore what the stories say about elders, about their role as guides, and about the nature of *both* rites of passage.

The Way Down Is the Way Up

Agony... is not denied to any man and...is given in strange ways to children.
— Flannery O'Connor[8]

MR. HEAD IS TAKING HIS TEN-YEAR-OLD grandson, who has been in his charge most of the boy's life, to Atlanta to teach him a lesson. The boy has an attitude, gives him lip, and needs to find out, once and for all, that "he was not as smart as he thought he was." With age, Mr. Head has "enter[ed] into that calm understanding of life that makes him a suitable guide for the young." He's up to the task, "entirely confident that he [can] carry out the moral mission of the coming day."

Things for Mr. Head, of course, go downhill from here. He oversleeps and is wakened by Nelson who is fully dressed and frying fatback for their breakfast. Though the grandfather succeeds in getting them to the junction in the woods where the train stops to let them board, in the rush to get off in Atlanta he leaves their lunch behind. During the walking tour of the city, he tries to keep the dome of the train station in sight; but when Nelson realizes that they are passing the same shops, he takes other turnings which eventually lead deep into a black neighborhood and leave the pair utterly lost.

Nelson asks a black woman for directions — under the circumstances, a courageous act that puts Nelson further ahead in their ongoing game of one-upmanship — and they learn there is hope: They can follow the streetcar tracks in the middle of the road back to the station. But are they walking in the right direction? It seems so, when their walking soon leads out of the black neighborhood. At this point Nelson, exhausted from hunger and walking, insists they stop.

The betrayal that is the central action at the heart of the story occurs after the boy falls asleep on the sidewalk. Mr. Head has decided "to teach [the] child a lesson he won't forget." For a time, hiding in the nearby alley, he just watches; but then, mindful that they have a train to catch, he kicks an empty garbage can to create a noise that will rouse the boy. Nelson starts awake, finds himself abandoned, and dashes down the street more quickly than his grandfather can chase him. When Mr. Head finds him three blocks away, Nelson has knocked over a woman who was carrying groceries; the woman is claiming he has broken her ankle and threatening "to call for an officer." A chorus of gathered supportive women denounce the "juve-nile deliquent." With the terrified boy now clinging to him, Mr. Head looks at the women "massed… to block his escape" and says:

> "This is not my boy," he said. "I never seen him before."

> The women dropped back, staring at him with horror, as if they were so repulsed by a man who would deny his own image and likeness that they could not bear to lay hands on him. Mr. Head walked on, through a space they silently cleared, and left Nelson behind. Ahead of him he saw nothing but a hollow tunnel that had once been the street.

This "hollow tunnel" is a symbolic allusion to Dante's *Inferno* — one of many that abounds throughout the story. At the beginning, Mr. Head is compared to "Virgil summoned in the middle of the night to go to Dante." The circuits the pair make around the train station are emblematic of a descent into hell as is the city's sewer system into which "a man could slide," Mr. Head explains to Nelson, "and be sucked along down endless pitch-black tunnels… and never [be] heard from again." The hell into which Mr. Head has been sucked is not some future place; it is here and now — and measurable with a tape measure. It is the very specific, unbridgeable 20 feet that now separate the two during their lost wanderings through the city.

> He could feel the boy's steady hate, traveling at an even pace behind him and he knew that (if by some miracle they escaped being murdered in the city) it would continue just that way for the rest of his life. He knew that now he was wandering into a black strange place where nothing was like it had ever been before, a long old age without respect and an end that would be welcome because it would be the end.

On the surface, O'Connor's story would seem to be about the *first passage* of life, where the elder-guide helps the initiate move from childhood/adolescence into adulthood. But the story, which "reverses a traditional pattern of initiation stories and has the elder instructor achieving more wisdom than the child initiate,"[9] is, in fact, a story of the *second passage* — and, therefore, like *The Inferno*, a *narrative of descent*.

It is Mr. Head, not Nelson, who is being initiated. But, in fact, you could make a strong argument that there are really not two separate characters here. "They were grandfather and grandson but they looked enough alike to be brothers." Jungians would say Nelson is Mr. Head's shadow side, and his developmental task is to *integrate* the "scowling" and "grinning" "ghosts" — the one full of "ancient wisdom" ("as if he knew everything already and would be pleased to forget it"), the other blithely unaware — which stare back at the pair from the windows of the train:

> [Nelson] turned his head to the glass. There he saw a pale ghost-like face scowling at him beneath the brim of a pale ghost-like hat. His grandfather, looking quickly too, saw a different ghost, pale but grinning, under a black hat.

One of my reasons in selecting the O'Connor story is because it contains a consummate dramatization of the havoc which *uninitiated old men* — I put this in italics, but maybe I need to repeat it — uninitiated old men, like Mr. Head, loose on the world — in the form of wars, predatory capitalism, and, in this story, the perpetuation of racism. A scene on the train captures exquisitely how racial prejudice is ingested by the young and the "sins of the father visited upon the son." It merits a careful, thoughtful reading and rereading.

When a "huge coffee-colored man" walks down the aisle of the train, Mr. Head grabs Nelson's arm and alerts him. After the man has passed, he asks Nelson:

> "What was that?"
>
> "A man."
>
> "What kind of a man?"
>
> "A fat man," Nelson said. He was beginning to feel that he had better be cautious.
>
> "You don't know what kind?"
>
> "An old man," the boy said and had a sudden foreboding that he was not going to enjoy the day.
>
> "That was a nigger," Mr. Head said and sat back… "I'd of thought you'd know a nigger since you seen so many when you was in the city on your first visit," Mr. Head continued. "That's his first nigger," he said to the man across the aisle.
>
> The boy slid down into the seat. "You said they were black," he said in an angry voice. "You never said they were tan. *How do you expect me to know anything when you don't tell me right?*" …He felt that the Negro had deliberately walked down the aisle in order to make a fool of him and *he hated him with a fierce raw fresh hate*; and also, he understood now why his grandfather disliked them.

If this is a *story of betrayal*, it is also, ultimately, a *story of redemption*. "Redemption" is a word with layers of meaning. For our purposes, it is enough if we take it to describe the attainment of some much-needed self-knowledge, the melting of the heart, and an unlooked for and undeserved reconciliation.

Mr. Head "had never known before what mercy felt like because he had been too good to deserve any." Though twice his age, he must arrive like Dante at that point where he can admit he's lost: "I'm lost!' he called.

'I'm lost and can't find my way and me and this boy have got to catch this train and I can't find the station. Oh Gawd I'm lost!'"

Only at this point can the miraculous and impossible happen. There are, as we witness in the powerful scene in the film *Gandhi*, "ways out of hell."[10] The unbridgeable distance between the two — the 20 feet that separate them as they wander lost through the city — *is* bridged. It is bridged inexplicably through what Martin Luther King called "the redemptive power of unmerited suffering" (symbolized in the story by the weathered statue of a black lawn jockey) and what Flannery O'Connor calls "the action of mercy."

> They stood gazing at the artificial Negro as if they were faced with some great mystery, some monument to another's victory that brought them together in their common defeat. They could both feel it dissolving their differences like an action of mercy.

At the end of the story, Mr. Head stands "appalled, judging himself with the thoroughness of God, while the action of mercy covered his pride like a flame and consumed it. He had never thought himself a great sinner before but he saw now that his true depravity had been hidden from him lest it cause him despair." If this language seems extreme, it must be read in light of the scene on the train and the injunction of Jesus that "whosoever shall scandalize one of these little ones that believe in me: it were better for him that a millstone were hanged about his neck and he were cast into the sea."[11]

As the Greeks knew long ago, it is only through suffering — that "agony, which is not denied to any man and... is given in strange ways to children" — only through the descent — that wisdom comes:

> *He who learns must suffer*
> *And even in our sleep pain that cannot forget*
> *Falls drop by drop upon the heart,*
> *And in our own despite, against our will,*
> *Comes wisdom to us by the awful grace of God.*[12]

Breaking the Rules — *Properly*

> *A man's heart is like a caged bird. When you dance, your heart sings... and then rises to heaven.*
>
> — *Monsieur Ibrahim*[13]

M*onsieur Ibrahim* is a period piece set in the 1960s in the Blue Road working-class district of Paris. Moses Schmidt has just turned 16 when we meet him and — with help from a kindly prostitute who works the bustling street in front of his apartment building — is about to get laid for the first time. He lives alone with his father who is suffering wounds from his abandonment by his wife. He not only neglects the boy (forgetting this milestone birthday, for example), but repeatedly shames him with disparaging comparisons to his absent older brother Paulie.

When the father loses his job, he abandons the boy to his own devices, leaving behind this note:

> Son, excuse me, I've left. I'm not cut out to be a father. Perhaps we'll meet again one day when you're a man... when I'm less ashamed, and you forgive me. I've left my money on the table with a list of people to contact. They'll take care of you. Goodbye.

In the meantime, a relationship has been developing between Momo and an unlikely ally, the older "Arab"[14] whose small grocery is across the street. We learn he is a Sufi (which is "not a disease," he assures Momo, but "a way of thinking. *Although, some ways of thinking are diseases too*"). In his role as guide to the young boy, Ibrahim showers on him a long litany of "survival tips": how to make paté from cat food that will pass muster with his father, how to water down the Beaujolais, how to smile to win the girls.

In writing about the role of grandparents — and, by extension, elders — John Sullivan identifies three tasks. The first is to "*Bless the Young*: Grandparents at their best see us in our unique core beauty. They see us as deeper than our actions; and, hence in their presence, we often become our better selves."[15] The affirmations from Ibrahim begin the work of repairing Momo's damaged ego.

> Momo: If I was like Paulie, Dad would love me.
> Ibrahim: How do you know? Paulie left. Maybe he hated your dad.
> Momo: You think so?
> Ibrahim: Why else would he leave?
> Momo: ... Did you know Paulie?
> Ibrahim: *I prefer you a hundred times. I prefer you a hundred times.*

A second task, according to Sullivan, is to "*Keep the Big Things Big and the Little Things Little*: Grandparents [know] the wisdom of 'This too shall pass' [and can reassure] the young who often stay stuck in the limited drama of the moment."[16] When the girl that Momo fancies dumps him for a competitor, he complains, trapped in the negative script: "There's always a Paulie eating me up inside." "It doesn't matter, Momo," Ibrahim tells him. "Your love for her is yours. It belongs to you. She rejects it, but she can't destroy it. She's just missing out on it." This too shall pass.

All this advice and attention comes tied in a package which to Momo, who has never experienced *unconditional love*, must at first be bewildering. Early in the film we see Momo pinching cans from the shelves of the grocery store. Some scenes later, a casual comment — "I have to make up for all the cans you pinch"— makes it clear the petty larceny has not gone unobserved by Ibrahim. Full of remorse, Momo promises, "I'll pay you back."

> Come here, Momo... Listen to me. You owe me nothing. If you have to steal, I prefer you do it in my shop. Look at me. You owe me nothing.[17]

His father gone, Momo is getting on just fine in the world, feeding and clothing himself and creatively financing his continuing sexual inquiry by selling off — five or six tomes at a time — his father's extensive library of Biblical exegeses. Then the police arrive. The news they bring is that his father has abandoned him in the most profound of ways... by committing suicide. The threat they bring is that, since he is under age and has no relatives, he must become the ward of the state. It is at this point in the film that Ibrahim legally adopts the boy as his son.

The final segment of the film is a road trip in which the two travel together (in a sporty red convertible that Ibrahim has bought) from Paris to Ibrahim's home in a small village in Turkey, where after an automobile accident, Ibrahim dies, leaving Momo another note — from his true father:

> I, Ibrahim Demirdji, hereby leave all my goods to Moses Schmitt, my son Momo, because he chose me as his father, and because I've given him everything I've learned in this life. *Now you too will know what's in my Koran*, Momo. It's all there is to know.

In the film, both the father and the shopkeeper give Momo advice. His father, for example, gives him a piggybank when he is very young: "You put the coin here," he demonstrates, "...in the slot." The boy takes the piggybank, turns it upside down, and rattles the coin around. "It can't come out," he protests.

> Father: Money's made to be saved, not spent.
> Momo: And when it's full?
> Father: When it's full, you're rich.

Sound first-half-of-life financial advice. First-half-of-life thinking — or, let us start to use the phrase, "first half of life *spirituality*" — helps us get along in the world. It provides us with necessary ethical moorings — discouraging murder, theft, dishonesty, promiscuity, and all the other "sins" covered by the last seven Commandments. In other instances, it may be *ethically neutral*, like the financial advice Momo's father gives him.[18] In the worst instances, it is soul-destroying, like the "tutorial" Mr. Head gives Nelson on the train. Part of the point is that first-half-of-life thinking doesn't seem to know the difference between life-affirming and life-denying advice.

Second half of life thinking — or, we might with more accuracy say, second-half-of life *loving* — is an invitation to inhabit a larger, more spacious world. John Sullivan captures something of what this means in the third "task" he assigns to grandparents (and elders, by extension), namely, to "*Encourage Creativity*: Grandparents… can be allies of the young by encouraging them to be daring, take risks, follow their dreams."[19] Yes, the world is larger in this way; but, more importantly, that larger world is *riddled with paradox*. Earlier, in quoting the advice which Ibrahim gives Momo after the girl he fancies dumps him, I omitted the important last two sentences:

> Your love for her is yours. It belongs to you. She rejects it, but she can't destroy it. She's just missing out on it. *What you give, Momo, is yours for good. What you keep is lost forever.*

Something as simple as a smile participates in this paradoxical character. Asked why he never smiles, Momo says he "can't afford to… Smiling is for the rich. I mean it's for happy people." "You're wrong," Ibrahim tells him. "*Smiling is what makes you happy.*" Echoes of a saying of the Zen Buddhist monk, Thich Nhat Hanh: "Sometimes your joy is the source of your smile, but sometimes your smile can be the source of your joy."

The Dance of Spirit in Later Life

The foundational paradox is this: We must "learn the rules" for this reason — *"so that you know how to break them properly."*[20] A primary task of later life is to move from a *religion of rules* to a *spirituality of the heart*. Not only were rules made to be broken; our salvation depends on it. "There is a crack in everything," the lyrics to the song "Anthem" tell us: *"that's how the light gets in."*[21]

Here is a point that I haven't made yet. Whether the initiate is an adolescent poised to enter adulthood or a midlife adult on the verge of elderhood, the guidance the elder-guide offers is always grounded in second-half-of-life wisdom. There are not two separate codes of knowledge; there is one trove of perennial wisdom. What Momo can understand at 16 is, of course, different from what the Englishman Basil — battered by an additional 20 years of life experience — can understand. But just as the teacher appears when the student is ready,[22] the seeds he or she plants will ripen in the fullness of time.

What Ibrahim does for Momo is to essentially serve as his "spiritual director." Like every good teacher, he gives Momo homework — research. After learning that Ibrahim is a Sufi, Momo looks the word up in one of his father's reference books (which he will later sell) and learns that it is a "mystical form of Islam [that] stresses inner religion" and is "opposed to legalism." "Legalism," he learns, refers to the "meticulous observance of the law."

He is drawn to the Sufi because of his joy — joy which is "the most infallible sign of the presence of God" (Teilhard de Chardin). He knows that his father's own brand of legalistic Judaism is joyless. Asked earlier by Ibrahim, "What does being Jewish mean to you?" "I don't know," he answers. "For my dad, it means being depressed all day."

"How do you manage to be happy?" he asks Ibrahim, who answers enigmatically, "I know what's in my Koran." He will repeat that same profession almost verbatim six other times in the film. Yet when Momo asks, "Should I read your Koran?," he gives another enigmatic reply: "If God wants to reveal life to you, he won't need a book." At the end of the film we learn that what is in Ibrahim's Koran is two pressed blue flowers.

During the road trip near the end of the film, Ibrahim imparts more life lessons. In Istanbul, he takes Momo to an Orthodox church, a Catholic church, and a Muslim mosque and *blindfolds* him, so he can open to these places of worship through his senses.

This course in comparative religion culminates with a stunning scene in which the two witness the dance of a group of whirling dervishes. The whole film has been building to this penultimate scene, and it is now that Ibrahim invites Momo to join the sacred dance:

> Ibrahim: I'll make you dance.
> Momo: You?
> Ibrahim: Yes, you must. Absolutely. A man's heart is like a caged bird. When you dance, your heart sings... and then rises to heaven. They spin around their hearts. God is there, in their hearts. It's like a prayer. They lose all their bearings, that burden we call balance. They become like torches. They burn in a blazing fire.

"Teach me to dance!"

> *And when you get the choice to sit it out or dance, I hope you dance.*[23]

WE HAVE LOOKED AT THREE narratives in which the figure of the elder appears. In all three, the elder plays the role of guide. In *Monsieur Ibrahim*, the rite of passage for the 16-year-old Momo is from adolescence into adulthood; the story is one of *ascent*, because the energy at this time of life follows the arc of ascent. In *Zorba the Greek*, the rite of passage for the 35-year-old Englishman — in this narrative of *descent* in which "the way down is the way up"— is from midlife into elderhood. The *sage* in both stories provides counsel that is grounded in a second-half-of-life wisdom — how to break the rules properly, how to welcome that "madness" that will free us, how to enter a larger, inclusive world.

In the remaining story, the elderly Mr. Head is a Lear-like figure — who being old, should have been wise.[24] He is a false guide to Nelson, visiting upon his young charge his own soul-destroying prejudice. The out-of-season rite of passage — all too common in a society that has forgotten the need for ceremonies of initiation and lacks sages who could guide them — which the story describes is his own attainment to self-knowledge which he can arrive at only through a painful descent.

"Teach me to dance," Basil says to Zorba, at the end of the film. How better to end this essay than with Zorba's response: "Did you say... 'dance'? Come on, my boy!"[25]

One of the [soul's] best-kept secrets, and yet one hidden in plain sight, is that the way up is the way down. Or, if you prefer, the way down is the way up... [It is] a secret, probably because we

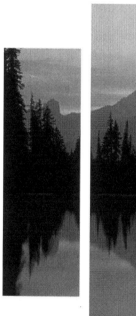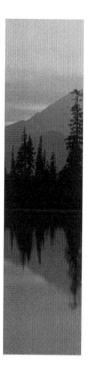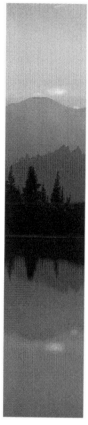

do not want to see it. We do not want to embark on a further journey if it feels like going down, especially after we have put so much sound and fury into going up.

— RICHARD ROHR

Construction Of Time

Old men and children are close
The young have just come
The old are soon going there
They can stand and watch all day
Watch men with hammer and bulldozer
A new building.

Old men on park benches and fishing piers
They don't say much
They don't have to
It's the young who talk

Old men and babies are quiet
Babies absorb it all
They cry if they hurt
Old men hurt and don't cry

They are between a world that rises
And one that falls
They have an agenda
Which is another way to
Say beginning middle and end

When I am one of the old men
I will take my stand
To watch the will of the world
I want to be in line

Waiting to see what the world's doing
I will have a button to push
To stop it if it moves too fast

The children and I can
Look for a while and
They won't have to grow up.
— Grady Bennett Myers, Jr.

This is a Call to Action

WHAT ARE YOU WAITING FOR?

by Darcy Ottey

to the baby boomer generation. Over the last five years, I have been blessed to sit in many cross-generational circles. I have attended "elder initiation ceremonies" with hundreds of guests. These opportunities have helped me understand better the challenges that face aging adults, and they have provided insight about what our society needs from folks as they age. I have been struck time and again by the hesitation of older people to claim the role of elder, either because of a fear of becoming old (and thus irrelevant) or a fear of being so audacious in claiming a wisdom they feel they lack.

I suppose my impatience is rooted in my youth. From my perspective, my generation and the generations that follow are inheriting a very challenged planet, and we need all the help we can get. So again: This is a Call to Action. If you're over 50, please step forward and fake it until you make it as an Elder.

What might that mean? Here are some of the things I've learned over the last five years.

Share your stories / share your wisdom

I HEAR RESISTANCE FROM MANY of you baby boomers to call yourselves elders, because you don't feel you've attained enough wisdom to qualify as an elder. It is as though you believe you need to know what you're doing to be an elder. But the challenge is that our cultural models for how to truly be an elder no longer exist, so how are you going to learn?

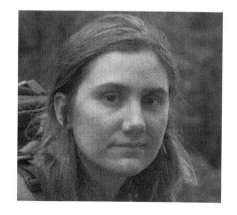

This is a perfect task for your generation; you've been doing exactly this — pushing the cultural edges — since you came along. You emerged into a world of values that you didn't share, and you pushed hard to create something new.

Throughout your teens, twenties, thirties, and beyond, your passion for creating new forms led to a lot of mistakes and failures. It's also led to a huge number of inspiring successes. Those of us coming into our prime adult life are grateful for both the new paths you've blazed — AND all the failures you had from which we can learn. We don't always know the questions to ask. We need your guidance! Please share it. You don't need to know what it means to be an elder. It's fine if you learn as you go. You'll make horrible blunders along the way. But hopefully by the time you're done, my generation will have a road map.

Give us space to lead and to make mistakes

IF YOU WANT MORE than that, I can tell you what I want personally. I don't know if it's shared by my peers, but I think it is. Being an elder is about giving up center stage and allowing those of us following in your footsteps to begin to take leadership. I often see a hesitation to step back among aging baby boomers. I believe that the root of this hesitation is fear of becoming irrelevant. But it's couched in very different clothing. Usually, it's dressed up in statements like, "I've been doing this for 30 years. I'll do it better than someone who's just learning. We want the work to be the best it can be, right?" That's all well and good — until one day you up and die. I realize that I have a lot to learn, and I'll stumble and make mistakes as I learn things that by now come naturally to you. Nonetheless, it'll be far easier for me to learn while you're here to answer questions and offer guidance.

I know that's a far more awkward role for you, because it means you don't really have anything to do. But I can tell you that if you open your time up to eldering, there will be plenty of young people banging down your door for guidance. And then your only task is to simply be.

Offer blessings

ONE OF THE GREATEST GIFTS you can offer as an elder is the act of blessing. When I reflect on the mentorship I received from Stan Crow, the founder of Rite of Passage Journeys and my mentor and elder for 18 years, his greatest contribution to me was that he blessed me. I inherited his organization from him, and he graciously stepped out of the way almost immediately, despite the fact that he had poured 25 years of blood, sweat, and tears into the program, and I clearly had absolutely no idea what I was doing. He let me lead, he let me make mistakes. And when I didn't know what to do, I would knock on his door. He would invite me in, give me a cup of tea, listen to me share my concerns and questions. And then he'd smile, and tell me I was doing a great job. He'd tell me that it sounded like I knew just what to do. He offered me his blessing, and it gave me an enormous amount of confidence. I believe that he made me a far stronger leader by doing this than by telling me what I should do — even if he probably had far better ideas than those I proposed.

When he died last year, and I couldn't ask him for his advice, I could still call on him to offer me a blessing. And I knew just what Stan's blessing sounded like.

Take care of yourself

Randy Morris, Director of Spiritual Studies at Antioch University Seattle, had a large public event to mark his 60th birthday and initiation into elderhood. One of his students, Elizabeth Zinda, was invited to speak for all of his students about what they would ask for him as he enters into his elder years. Elizabeth said many wise things. But the moment I will always remember was when she looked Randy straight in the eye, and said, "Take care of yourself. Take care of your body. Take care of your health. Because what we need most from you is that you're able to live as long as you can." This may be the most important principle of elderhood there is, and also likely the hardest.

Teach us how to care for you

Several years ago, at a large cross-cultural and cross-generational gathering, I watched as a woman my age stood up, walked across the room, and offered an older man a chair to sit in while he was speaking. She said "Excuse me, elder, I should know better than to let you stand there without offering you a seat. My apologies." He warmly accepted the seat.

I learned a lot from the younger woman in this encounter about what it means to confer respect upon our elders with simple, caring gestures of kindness. I learned a lot from the older man about accepting this kind of care and respect.

The situation could have gone differently. The older man could have said, "Thank you, I'm happy to stand," or said, "I can take care of myself." Thank goodness he didn't. Whenever an elder allows him or herself to be cared for, they offer a gift to the community. Personally, I find that when an older person is willing to accept small gestures of kindness from me, it makes me a kinder, more caring person in general. I feel better about myself, and more aware of the people around me.

I've observed this in how my husband related to his grandmother as well. She passed away last year, almost 90. What made me fall in love with him, more than anything, was watching the patient attentiveness he showed to his grandmother, helping her out of the car, holding an umbrella over her as we walked, doing small tasks around her apartment to make her life easier. When older people accept this kind of care with grace, it makes us all better people.

But I think many young people don't really know how to offer kindness, care, and true respect. Honestly, it's not something we're taught. So that's another place where elders can serve — by teaching us through both words and example how to care for you, and reinforcing our feeble attempts with "Thank you," smiles, and gentle suggestions.

Traditional cultures revered, and continue to revere, their elders as wisdom-keepers. But there is no roadmap left in our culture for what it means to be an elder. Similarly, younger generations have no roadmap for how to truly respect our elders and how to seek guidance from them. Yet there are many places to learn how to do this! Increasingly, organizations and communities around our country are creating opportunities for elders to hold a place of service. In addition, there are many organizations (like Rite of Passage Journeys) that offer programs to help folks think about what it is they have to offer in elderhood. There are creative aging Web sites and study groups. And probably, as you look around your block, there are young people just waiting for guidance and an older adult to take an interest in their lives.

Don't hesitate. Reach out today, and continue to make a difference in the world. Maybe, just maybe, your greatest contribution is still to come.

When I consider a spiritual book, I think of one that reminds me that I'm part of the great mystery that I'll never fully understand, yet always yearn to be part of. The book that greatly inspired my spiritual journey is *The Voice of the Earth* by Theodore Roszak. This book launched ecopsychology, which posits that "The Earth hurts, and we hurt with it." Roszak weaves together psychology, cosmology, and ecology to show that the Earth is alive, that people rely on it for all their complex levels of well-being, and that limiting pathways of mental healing to the human family alone is like studying the moon and saying you understand the universe. "The planet's umbilical cord," says Roszak, "links to us at the root of the unconscious mind." In this book, science and spirit, history and individual striving meet where the soul encounters the Earth.

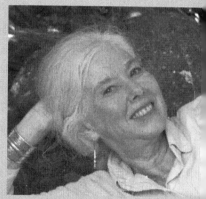

Trebbe Johnson

Trebbe Johnson is the author of *The World Is a Waiting Lover* and the founder of Radical Joy for Hard Times, a nonprofit organization devoted to finding and making beauty in wounded places. She leads workshops and journeys internationally that combine the mythic quest and the exploration of wisdom and insight through nature.

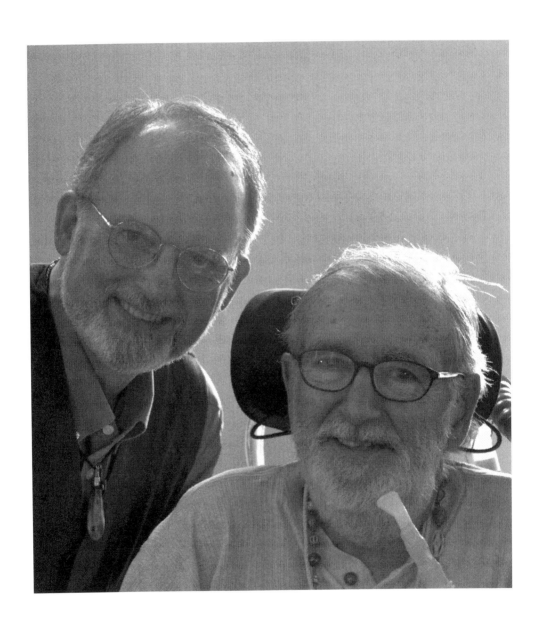

Honoring Our Elders

FRED LANPHEAR: EARTH ELDER

Fred Lanphear lived his life with great intentionality — about his career (his calling or vocation), his devotion to his family, and his role as elder.

He'd begun his career as an agronomist, a scientist convinced that modern industrial agriculture held the key to providing for future human needs. Slowly, however, his awareness of the harmful consequences of this mindset began to grow. The next phase of his life was service within a Christian service organization, the Institute of Cultural Affairs (ICA). He spent years in Africa and India, trying to foster community development by sharing the agricultural skills he'd learned.

After this work abroad had confirmed his sense of the importance of community development, Fred next turned his energies to helping found and grow an intentional cohousing community, Songaia, located on the outskirts of Seattle. After Songaia had become established, Fred took the next step, becoming a persuasive and effective advocate for the national intentional community movement, helping found the Northwest Intentional Community Association and serving on the board of the Fellowship for Intentional Community.

Up until now, community to Fred had meant the *human* community of family, friends, and associates. Then he read *The Dream of the Earth* by the cultural historian and ecotheologian Fr. Thomas Berry. Berry had argued that the old stories that have supported our cultures for millennia were no longer adequate for present conditions. The new story of evolution speaks of a profound *interrelatedness between all beings* in the cosmos within creative processes that have been operating over billions of years.

Community had to include all of the beings, living and nonliving, that inhabit planet Earth. Fred had devoted his life to nurturing the human community; now he sensed he was being called to something more: Given the needs of our time, living in the context of the "old stories" with their limited sense of community was no longer adequate.

Continuing to live his life intentionally, he chose the title Earth Elder to express his dedication to the "something more."

During these years an inner change had taken hold in Fred. As he approached his 60th birthday, he'd felt a need to mark and celebrate his passage into old age. He created a yearlong program for himself: traveling to Rhode Island to reconnect with family members and with the land and sea of his youth; creating a "mythological quilt" that depicted the primary involvement of each decade of his life; and undertaking a four-day vision quest. He then felt a renewed sense of calling and commitment to devote his remaining years to fostering the growth of communities that helped reconnect the human community with the natural world. Over the next decade, Fred's sense of his mission as elder grew, and by his 70th birthday he'd arrived at a deeper understanding: Becoming an elder meant becoming an elder for the Earth — becoming an *Earth Elder*.

What did being an elder mean to Fred? In traditional societies, the elder is one who is able to draw upon years of experience to provide guidance to the community. For Thomas Berry, elders are the storytellers who remind the community how it came into being and how it has survived the great challenges of the past. These stories bind the community together and provide the members with their sense of meaning and participation in the great community of existence.

For Fred, being an Earth Elder required he devote himself to three activities: *learning*, *living*, and *mentoring*.

"Learning the Great Story" meant learning a new story that differs from traditional stories of creation in several important ways. In the Great Story, the universe has been evolving and continues to evolve. The future of evolution and of continued life on Earth hinges on the choices and activities of the human community. Humans are deeply interdependent with all other members, living and nonliving, of the Earth community. A prime factor in our "fitness" to survive is our ability to forge mutually enhancing relationships — cooperation rather than competition.

"Living the Great Story" meant coming personally into a sustainable relationship with the processes of the planet. In Fred's cohousing community, many members strive to live in a manner that is conscious of the consequences of their choices for the larger Earth community. Earth and her systems are viewed as sacred, to be accorded reverence and to be celebrated. A labyrinth and peace garden are concrete manifestations of this sense, and Songaia members also celebrate the natural seasons of the planet, the solstices and equinoxes.

The final dimension, "Mentoring," meant not only being present to younger members of Songaia, but also helping the larger community find ways to celebrate the Great Story. He was inspired by a ritual called the Cosmic Walk, through which one is invited to reflect on the variety of gifts that have come into existence during the course of evolution. Fred led people in the ritual on a number of occasions, and one of his final gestures was to bequeath the Cosmic Walk materials to members of the Earth Elder study group, with instructions to "Tell the Story!"

After Fred was diagnosed with ALS, sensing that the terminal disease left him only a couple of years to live, the intentionality that had characterized so much of his life intensified: He invited members of Songaia, family members, and other friends to share his final journey. As the illness progressed, Fred accepted his neighbors' care graciously, freely sharing his feelings about his steadily progressing disability and its implications.

Until his final passing, Fred Lanphear, Earth Elder, dedicated himself to the challenge laid down by Pierre Teilhard de Chardin in a quote that Fred loved: "The task before us now, if we would not perish, is to shake off our ancient prejudices and rebuild the Earth."

— Jim Clark

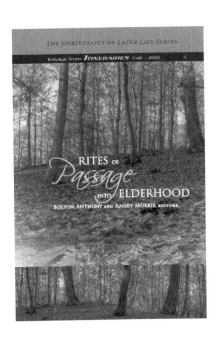

Rites of Passage into Elderhood

2011 Fall issue of Itineraries: Selections and Supplements

Earth Elder Initiation (NEW)
    by Randy Morris, Contributing Editor 195

Dreams and Elder Initiations
    by Harry R. Moody 205

Markers in the Stream
    by John G. Sullivan 215

Earth Elder Initiation

by **Randy Morris** with **Frost Freeman**

> *The time is ripe for elders to reclaim their rightful role of speaking for Earth and future generations.*
> — Fred Lanphear

A REVOLUTION OF ELDERS IS TAKING PLACE. Older people are accepting the responsibility to gather together in council and community to consider new visions for the role of elder in our culture. As conscious elders, some are choosing to step into this role by preparing themselves psychologically and spiritually through a rite of passage ceremony into elderhood. Of course, in past ages, elder initiation ceremonies were woven into the fabric of the culture, but in our current mainstream culture, we have lost the thread of these ceremonies. How can we revive the tradition of elder initiation in a culture that has forgotten its roots?

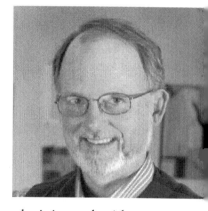

In past ages, new elders were chosen by initiated elders to undergo a rite of passage. But in a culture with few initiated elders, how does one get chosen? According to the principles of conscious eldering, a person of a certain age must choose to "heed the call" to eldership. This call is archetypal in nature, meaning that it springs from the instinctual, animal body of a human being who is in touch with themselves and with a "sacred other." It can be discerned in dreams, visions, strong emotions of grief and joy, synchronicities, epiphanies, and other manifestations of the unconscious, what the great ecotheologian Thomas Berry calls the "spontaneities" of the earth. To be able to perceive this call and respond to it requires that one be conscious of the very possibility of a "sacred other" and attentive to the voices of the more-than-human world. To be conscious in this way is to be spiritual, because it requires the ability to perceive, through heart-based capacities of intuition and feeling, the will of "unseen powers" at work both within the human psyche and the earth itself. This is one reason that conscious aging encourages encounters with the natural world where silence, solitude, and reflection open one's soul to the voices of the earth. In principle, the ability to perceive the call to elderhood is the birthright of every human being who is consciously engaging the life cycle with integrity and meaning.

To become a conscious elder requires that one experience a calling. But then what? How does one answer the call? Here is where the importance of modern elder initiation ceremonies becomes apparent. Initiation ceremonies are transformative rituals that have the power to reorient the individual will around a new set of values. While there are many different sets of values around which any elder initiation may be organized, an Earth Elder initiation espouses three specific values.

First, an Earth Elder recognizes that we are living in the time of a "Great Turning" when the future of the planet is in peril and human beings are called to serve the life-affirming powers of the earth. As Thomas Berry said, "The glory of the human has become the desolation of the earth; the desolation of the earth has become the destiny of the human." An Earth Elder is able to recognize the role that his or her own destiny is to play in the larger destiny of the human species.

Second, Earth Elders are aware of the "Universe Story" that tells of a new cosmological origin myth, beginning with the great "flaring forth" and evolving through the eons of life on earth to produce the unique gift of human consciousness. One implication of this new story is that human beings are now cocreators in the ongoing development of life on this planet. Without the cooperation of human beings, the trajectory of life on this planet will be tragically altered.

A third value of Earth Elders is a profound awareness of the "partnership of generations" that exists among the spirits of ancestors who have come before us, human beings who are alive in the present and the spirits of those generations yet to be born, generations who are counting on those of us who are alive today to make their lives possible. The capacity to experience the yearning of future generations requires a sensitivity to what the Gaian teacher Joanna Macy calls "deep time." These three values — the Great Turning, the Universe Story, and the Partnership of Generations — provide the core images around which an Earth Elder initiation is organized.

So what does an Earth Elder initiation look like? I am reminded of a principle of ritual spoken to me many years ago by another mentor, Stan Crow. He said, *"We're going to do this ritual the same way they've been doing it for ten thousand years: We're going to make it up as we go along!"* Of course, there are certain principles of ritual design that exist in every ceremony. There is the moment of separation in which we depart from the everyday world and step into another world characterized by imagination and longing. In this liminal space, various ritual gestures are made to assist the initiate in their encounter with sacred powers. And then the initiate returns to the everyday world with an elixir or gift to share with their community, thus encouraging the community to embrace new life. Having witnessed several Earth Elder initiations, and in the interests of encouraging many, many more, I would like to describe one such initiation ritual that took place recently in my community.

An Earth Elder Initiation

Separation — Frost is a 65-year-old woman who has lived a rich life of service in her community. Among her many activities, she serves as an elder for youth participants who return from a vision quest. She listens attentively to their stories and mirrors to them the rich messages contained in their experience. Last year she experienced a "call" to undergo an Earth Elder initiation. At first, she resisted this call. It was just too much attention to call to herself. Who was she to declare herself an Earth Elder? In this early stage of her initiatory process, she experienced a great deal of "ritual tension," a sure sign that she was on the right path. She writes in her journal:

> Mid-June: For 12 hours I've been looking out at the bay and where it meets the inlet, sitting in a driftwood-and-old-curtain sun shelter. I could say I am preparing for my coming elderhood initiation/celebration, but I could also say I don't know what I'm doing. I brought things to write and draw, and a couple fruit jars of water. I thought I'd do a lot of uninterrupted thinking and writing. It's been more like uninterrupted not-thinking. I'm amazed I can not-think for so long, and hope it's a positive sign. I was here at first light, watched the shadows turn, as if I'm sitting in a sundial, and now the sun and the western mountains are getting closer together. Suddenly the shelter falls apart around me. Well, I guess that's a sign! I pack up and go home. Next day I am full of energy.

> Late June: Fear, fear, fear, fear, fear. I keep alternating my gladness and excitement about this coming event with dread and anxiety. Fear seems to have a full closet of guises. These are the two that keep coming up so hard. My heart beats harder, my eyes close with dread. Will this be too "out there"? Will some old friends never … Should I be doing this in front of virtually everybody I know and love? Sometimes it doubles me over. Later, another aspect surfaces: I am dying to who I have been, and am becoming

not someone else, but another version of my true self. Oddly enough, knowing that leaves me calmer than the other fears. Still, the ego who rents out part of my mind is freaking out about it, "reasoning" with me while fanning the flames of the dread and anxiety. Back and forth, back and forth...

But after a deep conversation with a friend who reminded her that she was not doing this ceremony for herself alone, but for the sake of her whole community and the earth, she felt encouraged. Just after that talk, she took a walk in a nearby city park during which she encountered two owls in a cedar tree in the middle of the day, a very rare natural event that made her feel that her calling to become an Earth Elder was being blessed by the more-than-human world. She called together a group of friends to form a "wisdom circle" to help her design her ceremony, and she committed to a date in August for her Earth Elder Initiation. She writes:

Late July: I have been going through every photograph I own, and there are thousands. Some are for the 20-minute slide presentation of the path my life has gone; the rest will be for displaying in a special place for the celebration: other lifetime photos, ancestor pictures, teachers who have been important to me. Velda has offered to make me a garment to wear for it. I don't know what it will be like. The circle of friends who are putting their time and hearts into bringing all this about let me know that I'm not in charge of it now, and that I will not know everything that's going to happen. Randy and I have lunch and spend a lot of time talking about all this: fears, practicalities, being between two worlds, what being an elder might mean, how this event will affect other people besides myself... We walk in the park and find two owls, in full daylight, sitting about 6 feet above us. They spend quite a long time with us. You can only feel grateful for that, and things that go beyond words.

Early August: My "wisdom circle" meets. They give me tasks to do for the coming day. One is to be able to state my intentions for the rest of my life; in a few words, not goals, but guiding intentions. Second, to decide on three things that I would be willing to let go of once I cross the threshold of elderhood, and to make some artistic representation of each one that can then be burnt, buried, torn, etc. and to recognize what could emerge in their stead. Third, once I have crossed the threshold and been accepted into the elder circle, to have some words to say — wisdom that I'd like to share from my new place. It feels good to have some direction.

Day Before, August 24: I have everything ready. When I look out the window in the 6 am fog, a coyote scents the air. Oh man! What does this mean? It turns and goes the way it has come and slips into the woods. Several of us are at the Garden Club early, to start decorating. Sara and Zhalee work long, hard, and sincerely, and Roseanna helps with the baby and more ideas. I am again so touched by what all are putting into this. Velda brings my dress. It's beautiful! Full of greens, silk and cotton, with hand-beaded neck and moonstones sewn along a crocheted cord "path" in front. My son arrives from Minnesota, bringing his cousins from Seattle, Raksha and Sarah. Raksha draws out a henna design she has made for me, onto my arms and hands. I love having them overnight.

Morning of: The youngers go to help decorate some more, and will stay there. I am alone. Suddenly all the fear comes up again in a slightly different guise; the dread has been mostly gone for a couple weeks; this is sheer physical fear, fizzy bloodstream, dizzy legs, breathing not matching heartbeat any more. I do what I can. Velda returns, and helps. We go.

Initiation — Frost's initiation ceremony took place in a beautiful rustic setting: a garden club meeting room that had been decorated with flowers and filled with pictures and artifacts of her life. She invited about 40 friends and family members, most of whom had no idea what an elder initiation was. The "wisdom circle" that helped Frost design the ceremony made sure that there was an element of surprise in the ritual. Frost knew that the program would begin with an invocation of the spirits of the seven directions and various blessings by her community members. She knew she would tell her life story in a 20-minute slide show, describing how the key turning points in her life could be re-mythologized as preparation for her elderhood. And she knew that after a closing song, she and all of the guests would retire outside, while the wisdom circle members rearranged the room for the heart of the initiation ceremony. Frost was asked to prepare in advance three ritual gestures. First, she was asked to be able to state in concise terms her intentions for becoming an elder. Second, she was asked to create symbols for three things she was prepared to lay down and sacrifice before she entered the elder circle. Furthermore, she was asked to be able to name the new gift she would be able to pick up in the vacuum created by her sacrifice. And third, she was asked to prepare an "elder speech" that she would address to her community upon her recognition as an Earth Elder. The rest of the ceremony was meant to be a mystery to her, so that the spontaneities of her mythic consciousness could be invoked.

When members of the community were called back to the room, it had been arranged as a spiral leading to an archway. On the other side of the arch were six chairs for six elders — three women and three men. Each member of the community was asked to write down the date of their first encounter with Frost and to arrange themselves in chronological order along the spiral. Once this spiral was complete, the ritual began with the six elders speaking out loud amongst themselves, wondering who they would need to call from the spirit world to assist in the initiation of this Earth Elder. They decided that they would need Crone, the third member of the sacred manifestation of the Great Mother — Maiden, Mother, and Crone. And so they called for Crone to enter, and there she was, dressed in diaphanous blue robes, ready to be of service. The elders consulted themselves again and agreed that they would need to call on the spirit of Death itself to be present, since the awareness of death is so integral to the wisdom of an Earth Elder. So they called on Death, and out of an adjoining room swept a dark figure in black robes, rhythmically swaying and ready to join the ritual. With the scene set, the elders called out to Frost, and through the windows we could see her striding up to the door, resplendent in her ritual clothes and ready to enter the room. In Frost's own words:

> Zhalee comes outside to conduct me to the doorway. This is what I see. Heavy rope forms a spiral path to the center, where a threshold stands, on the other side of which are seated six elders. The room is dim, lit by candles and twilight. All guests are seated along this path, in the order in which they met me in my life. The Crone meets me at the door, and by this time, I'm not thinking, remembering, or relating. Death is crouched on the other side of the door. They say things. We are all in Someplace Else now, a place between two worlds. If I answer, or move, it's from a much older or more timeless aspect of me. My day-to-day self is not there. I am asked my intentions, and speak them: Aliveness; to increase my skills of mind, heart, and spirit; to make myself more visible as a mentor, teacher, counselor; and to invest in my curiosity. I have a basket and am invited to move along the spiral path toward the threshold of elderhood. As I go past my loved ones, they put into the basket notes of encouragement, thanks, blessing. Finally, at the threshold, I am asked what three things I am willing to leave behind.

For the past few months, ever since she was given this assignment by her wisdom circle, Frost had been thinking about what three things she would lay down, and what she would pick up. For each sacrifice, she created a handmade artistic representation. Here is what she said:

1. I let go of leftover SELF CRITICISM, even to condemnation. I know ways to do this, and as I do, the container that held the destructive is transformed to a container that holds the constructive: a power, a medicine bag that I now have the right to wear, for a lighter, more effective energy.
2. I let go of the belief that visible is vulnerable, INVISIBLE is invulnerable. This notion works well as a tool in the bag, but not as a way of being. I'm willing to be visible more often, and in contact with the world.
3. I let go of too much ALONENESS. I can offer great friendship and still maintain healthy boundaries, uncover seeds of new growth.

Once she lay down these three encumbrances and picked up their medicine, Death stepped forward and blessed them. Death was then asked to take her rightful place among the order of things. She went to the other side of the elders, opposite the threshold, and sat in an honored chair. Frost approached the edge of the threshold. Crone invited her, of her own free will, to step across. Frost paused, considered, and stepped across. She was greeted by Crone and gifted with Crone's own shawl. At that point, three women elders came forward and gifted her with a "universe story" necklace that they had made for her. Each bead and shell represented some aspect of the universe story, something that could inspire Frost, and draw her into balance and wisdom. Then the male elders stepped forward to present Frost with a decorated "beaver-hewed" wooden staff that had been blessed with waters from the healing springs of Lourdes, France. She was then invited to sit in a sacred chair, and the whole community of guests and elders gathered around her, touching her shoulders, head, arms, and knees. Those who could not reach her were invited to touch someone who was touching her until a web of interlocking hands and hearts were formed. Together, they chanted four long OM's as the elder blessings of her community were spiritually transmitted into Frost's soul. When it was over, Frost stood up as an initiated elder, and spoke to us from that place. In a firm voice, she said:

> I encourage you to do two things: honor your own life, and value happiness. I didn't say indulge your ego; think about all it took to come together and bring you here, now. How do you mean to spend that? How much time do you think you have? Make it good!
>
> And cultivate happiness. For centuries, we've been taught to put it last. Yet if you cultivate real happiness, you're healthier, with stronger immunities, more contentment and gratitude, true friends, you work better, and get led into finer adventures.
>
> But what about all the world problems? You'll be far stronger if you have what I just described. The world will never be saved by fear and starvation of the heart and soul. Honor your own life. And cultivate happiness.

With this climactic elder speech, the ceremony was nearly complete. Another elder led the group in a sound of joy, the directions were released, and instructions were given to prepare the potluck that was to follow. The ceremony was done.

Return — One of the most difficult aspects of any earth-centered ritual is the reincorporation phase. Without an intact culture to mirror the transformations that individuals undergo, it is hard to maintain the changes, and many initiates are tempted to regress into old patterns. Fortunately, Frost's wisdom circle was so energized by the work of preparing her ceremony, they wanted to keep meeting on a regular basis to consider further aspects of elder initiations and to serve as a support for other elders in the community. This was a good reminder that we don't consciously choose to be an Earth Elder for ourselves alone. The whole community benefits as the ties that bind are strengthened through heartfelt and intentional communal actions.

Two weeks after the initiation, Frost writes:

> The first day I only rested, alone. The next day I was moved to speak to a friend about a concern I had, and spoke AS an Earth Elder — a surprise to me, since I wasn't used to thinking in that term. I felt confident, and also aware that what I was saying wasn't "done" yet. I needed to get to a more useful place with my feelings and thoughts. Other days: I rest a lot! I try to think through what I'd like, and get stuck. What's up?? We (the circle) have a meeting scheduled to debrief, talk about how it was for us all.

I find myself saying I seem to get stuck in what I want to "get done," and am no longer sure what I WANT to do. There is a difference between the two, and I'm becoming aware of it. What a mystery! Something is trying to arise in me that's in line with my intentions and shared wisdom of that day: it has to do with curiosity, aliveness, cultivating happiness, etc., and I have a feeling, doing things without knowing entirely why I'm doing them. "If you build it, they will come." That covers a lot deeper and wider ground than setting goals. Meanwhile, the rest of the circle has been so deep into the whole process that when it's suggested that we might keep meeting as a wisdom circle for each other, there's a lot of agreement. The Youngers wonder whether it would be an elder circle they wouldn't be part of, but we quickly decide that we want these Youngers in it. It will help keep the elders with "fresh water" coming in to our thinking, and it will help "raise" the Youngers as they become elders.

Frost finally came to understand the significance of consciously choosing the role of Earth Elder:

This was intended to be more far-reaching than one person's celebration of life. We hoped to make clear to people that they had choices about how they lived and aged, many more choices than they realized. It has even gone beyond that, and we're truly on a continuing journey now!

We know that an initiation ceremony does not automatically transform the initiate into the full wisdom of an Earth Elder. There are many stages of learning yet to come. But it does serve to orient the initiate in their lifespan and set them on a path to wisdom that is recognized and blessed by their community. By all accounts, Frost's Earth Elder initiation ceremony was a great success. Of course, it was only one way of designing it. As we experiment with a revival of elder recognition ceremonies in a diverse and pluralistic culture, there is no single "right way." Much of the joy of the revival is in the design process itself, as the initiate and their beloved community talk and plan and play together. In this way, meaning is generated within the community itself and radiates out from there. If you were to call together your "wisdom circle" and plan your own Earth Elder initiation ceremony, how would *you* do it? As we pave the way for a "Revolution of Earth Elders," it is good to remember Fred Lanphear's call: "*The time is ripe for elders to reclaim their rightful role of speaking for Earth and future generations.*"

Well into the "second journey," my favorite spiritual books now address this profound time of life, and one in particular holds the strongest magic for me — *The Measure of My Days*, by Jungian analyst Florida Scott-Maxwell. I have more underlinings, scraps of paper, and paper clips embedded in this little volume than any other book on the aging shelf. I love to quote from its jumble of pithy declarations because this lady speaks with the intensity, courage, and clarity of the initiated. Writing in her 80's, deep in the transformational fires of aging, she says nearly everything I know to be true.

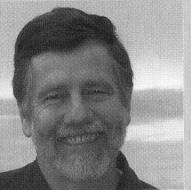

John C. Robinson

"I often want to say to people, 'You have neat, tight expectations of what life ought to give you, but you won't get it… Life does not accommodate you, it shatters you. It is meant to, and it couldn't do it better. Every seed destroys its container or else there would be no fruition.'"

John C. Robinson, Ph.D., D.Min., is a clinical psychologist with a second doctorate in ministry, an ordained interfaith minister, and the author of seven books on the interface of psychology and spirituality. His recent works include *The Three Secrets of Aging*; *Bedtime Stories for Elders: What Fairy Tales Can Teach Us About the New Aging*; and *What Aging Men Want: Homer's Odyssey as a Parable of Male Aging*. You can learn more about John at johnrobinson.org.

Dreams and Elder Initiations

by Harry R. Moody

"Is this all there is?" Peggy Lee asks in her famous song. Whether we have fulfilled our hopes in life, or realized that we never will, the question is still the same. "Is this all there is?"

That question invites us to begin a journey. It is the Call, the first of what I have described as the "five stages of the soul" in which the Call is followed by Search, Struggle, Breakthrough, and Return.[1] Though this initial invitation may come to us at any point in our lives, in later life it often comes with particular power and urgency.

The Call is an *awakening*, the moment when this inward dimension we call soul comes to life — that moment when we "come to ourselves" and ask the perennial questions: Who am I? Where am I going? What is this life all about? These questions prove painful because, as James Hollis puts it, by midlife what we have become — the strong ego we have built — is frequently our chief obstacle to listening to the Call.

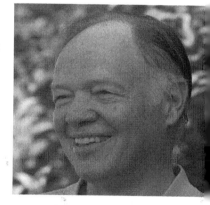

The inner voice demands to be heard — demands we begin the journey. Jung warns us of the price we pay if we ignore the invitation: "Only the man who can consciously assent to the power of the inner voice becomes a personality." Everything around us, however, conspires to keep us from hearing this "still small voice." We avoid looking inside ourselves because:

> Looking in will require of us great subtlety and great courage — nothing less than a complete shift in our attitude to life and to the mind. We are so addicted to looking outside ourselves that we have lost access to our inner being almost completely. We are terrified to look inward, because our culture has given us no idea of what we will find (Sogyal Rinpoche).

In ancient Shamanic traditions, the Call was recognized as an opening to initiation into the world of the spirits; this Call to initiation would often come through our dreams. The potential shaman who hears the call through his dreams ignores it at his peril: "Most shamanic traditions take the position that refusal to follow the call will result in a terrible accident, a life-threatening sickness, or insanity" (Stanley Krippner).

Do we dismiss this warning as just an ancient superstition? Or is it an all-too-accurate description of what happens when an entire culture, a global civilization, ignores the invitations of the soul seeking actualization? Today, as we see the world around us plunged in such collective insanity, we must wonder: How many around us have ignored the Call or dismissed its message? How many have ignored their dreams?

The Cry

THE GREAT JEWISH THEOLOGIAN Martin Buber begins his book *Between Man and Man* by telling about one of his own dreams, a classic dream of the Call. This dream came to him again and again, sometimes after an interval of years. In the dream he finds himself in a "primitive" world, in a vast cave or a mud building, or "on the fringe of a gigantic forest whose like I cannot remember having seen." Perhaps this "gigantic forest" is the same "dark wood" where Dante found himself at the beginning of his own spiritual journey. Here is Martin Buber's dream:

> The dream begins in very different ways, but always with something extraordinary happening to me, for instance, with a small animal resembling a lion-cub (whose name I know in the dream but not when I awake) tearing the flesh from my arm and being forced only with an effort to loose its hold. The strange thing is that this first part of the dream story, in the duration as well as the outer meaning of the incidents, always unfolds at a furious pace as though it did not matter. Then suddenly the pace abates: I stand there and cry out.

Buber goes on to tell us that, in terms of waking consciousness, he might suppose that his cry could be joyous or fearful, depending on interpretation. But when he remembers the dream in the morning, "the cry" is "neither so expressive nor so various." Instead, he remembers that "each time it is the same cry, inarticulate but in strict rhythm, rising and falling, swelling to a fullness which my throat could not endure were I awake…" The cry becomes a song, and "when it ends my heart stops beating."

> But then, somewhere, far away, another cry moves towards me, another which is the same, the same cry uttered or sung by another voice. Yet it is

not the same cry, certainly no echo of my cry but rather its true rejoinder, tone for tone, not repeating mine… so much so, that mine, which at first had to my own ear no sound of questioning at all, now appear as questions, as a long series of questions, which now all receive a response.

A dream like this cannot be translated into rational discourse: "The response is no more capable of interpretation than the question. And yet the cries that meet the one cry that is the same do not seem to be the same as one another. Each time the voice is new." Though the rational mind cannot grasp the meaning of this Cry, Buber still comes away from the dream with a sense of certitude: "A certitude, true dream certitude comes to me that now it has happened. Nothing more. Just this, and in this way —- now it has happened."

Martin Buber had this dream over and over again, until the last time just two years before he spoke about it in his book. Of the last instance of the dream, he wrote: "At first it was as usual…my cry died away, again my heart stood still. But then there was quiet. There came no answering call. I listened, I heard no sound." Buber, surprised by this absence, waits, in vain, for the response. But then something happened to him, a change of awareness, as if his senses had suddenly become magnified. "And then, not from a distance but from the air round about me, noiselessly, came the answer." Rather, the answer was already there, was present even before his cry: "When I laid myself open to it, it let itself be received by me." What he received at that moment he received "with every pore of his body." Once again, he experienced profound certainty, "pealing out more than ever, that now it has happened."

What Martin Buber has so beautifully described in this dream is the powerful, overwhelming reality of the Call. It is what the poet Rilke speaks of (in the *Duino Elegies*) when he tells of listening to the call of "the Angel" and realizing that to have lived on Earth, "To have been here once, if only for this once, can never be cancelled." In essence, it has happened. The Call is a moment of certainty, but not a dogmatic conclusion that can be put into words. On the contrary, it is a hunger for the Infinite.

Rilke put it beautifully in his *Letters to a Young Poet*: "Be patient toward all that is unsolved in your heart and try to love the questions themselves. Do not now seek the answers, which cannot be given you because you would not be able to live them. And the point is to live everything. Live the questions." The Call, then, is different from some "religious experience," or any sort of "conversion" that gives us clear or definitive conclusions. Quite the contrary. The Call is an encounter with emptiness, with our own deepest questions, now no longer experienced as doubt but as certainty: It has happened.

But to listen to the Call we must learn to listen to an Inner Voice.

The Old Men in the Cave

INITIATION INTO ELDERHOOD need not come only in later life. On the contrary, in world mythology, we find repeated pairing between the young hero and a hero who represents the Elder Ideal. The following is the dream of a young man who was seeking direction in his life. He had gone alone to camp on Mt. Shasta in California where he was practicing nightly "dream incubation," a custom familiar to the ancient Greeks. On the fifth night on the mountaintop he had the following dream:

> I am in a cave with a group of old men. They are drinking water from an old bowl that is being passed around. As the bowl comes closer towards me I realize that this must be a dream. An old man with dark skin and dark hair sitting next to me hands me the bowl. I take it and drink the water. I suddenly hear a humming sound and as I look up the men have disappeared and a beautiful white deer is walking in the light in the far distance. I awake feeling ecstatic.

The dreamer considered this lucid dream to be an initiatory experience. Apart from the dreamer's individual psychological associations, key features of this dream are important for understanding the place of dreams over the life course.

In every respect, "The Old Men in the Cave" is a dream of initiation during youth. The dreamer goes alone out into the wilderness, as would be the custom for a Native American shaman seeking dream initiation. Among the Plains Indians the dream was treated as a significant event, occurring on different planes of reality. Thus, among such groups the "vision quest" was also known as "crying for a dream" and was found especially among the Lakota. Among the Iroquois it was understood that the spirit world could communicate with individuals through these "Big Dreams." The Mohawk word *atetshents* means, simply, "one who dreams," the same word used for a shaman or healer. A Big Dream could be a healing for the whole community, conveying revelations or warnings to be heeded.

Though the young man who dreamed "The Old Men in the Cave" was not a Native American, the condition and the imagery of his dream have lessons well beyond him. The psychological journey into the self is, in many respects, a path toward aloneness. Each of us must learn to be alone with ourselves. The journey into the wilderness is also a passage into an unknown world, to discover something in us that is wild and untamed. The dreamer here has actually gone to a mountaintop in order to incubate his dream; and the mountaintop, too, is a significant symbol: It is the point where Earth touches heaven. Recall that Moses went to the top of Mt. Sinai to receive revelation, and Muhammad went into a cave atop Mount Hira, where he received the revelation of the Quran. Yet the setting of this dream has another curious feature. It is not only on the mountaintop but also in an opposite direction: that is, downward, into a cave, as if suggesting, in the words of Heraclitus, "The way up and the way down are the same."

Caves symbolize what is deepest and oldest in the psyche. "Before humans built shelters, the earliest sacred places were caves," writes A. T. Mann: "The connection of cave to underworld remains a primary ancestral memory for us, and thus, caves remain formidable places." Joseph Campbell says: "The cave has always been the scene of initiation, where the birth of the light takes place. Here as well is found the whole idea of the cave of the heart, the dark chamber of the heart, where the light of the divine first appears."

The oldest art works of humanity — the cave art at Lascaux or the even older cave of Chauvet in France — are cave drawings from our remote ancestors. Cave dwelling evokes a primordial condition which can be understood as the context for this dream. The dreamer at first is not alone in this cave but is with a group of old men, as if to suggest that the process of initiation itself is a connection between youth and age. As in the ritual of the Eucharist, in "The Old Men in the Cave" a bowl is passed around and, just as the dreamer is about to drink, the dream becomes lucid. The image of an old man with "dark skin" and "dark hair" suggests an element of darkness or shadow belonging to the dreamer, who has now drunk from the initiatory bowl. From that moment on the old men in the dream disappear, and the dreamer is once again alone. The circle of aloneness is complete. As philosopher Alfred North Whitehead once remarked, religion is what each of us does with our aloneness.

The cave drawings at Lascaux and Chauvet depict magical animals, and in "The Old Men in the Cave" the dreamer now sees another magical animal: the "white deer walking in the light in the far distance." This vision of an illuminated animal symbolizes the distance this dreamer has already traveled and must still travel in the process of initiation. The dreamer has now been granted a holy vision, and he wakes up ecstatic. The word *ek-stasis*, in Greek means, literally, "standing outside oneself," as this dreamer has gone outside himself.

"The Old Men in the Cave" is the dream of a young man seeking guidance. But where can youth find guidance today? In a society like ours where age is devalued, young people are left adrift. Not surprisingly, they crave some kind of initiation or viable path into adulthood. Because we lack any journey into the wilderness, or a genuine ritual for reconciling aloneness within society, we end up forcing young people to behave in ways disconnected from the adult world and from the self they might become. And so they join gangs to find solidarity and a viable path to adulthood. The image of the elders in "The Old Men in the Cave" expresses a longing for such guidance and direction in life — a longing that too often remains unfulfilled.

This challenge of initiation is not limited to young people. At every transitional or "liminal" stage of life we need guidance. "There persists in all of us, regardless of gender, an archetypal need to be initiated," as Jungian analyst Anthony Stevens writes, even though "our culture no longer provides rites of initiation, except in training members of the armed forces and providing examinations for students." So we turn to stories, myths, fairy tales, and dreams that respond to our hunger for a "rite of passage" that will help us move during critical or transitional points in the life course — marriage, death of a parent, and so on — to the next stage of life.

Meeting the Sage

> I am sitting in a pastoral setting, watching a strange event take place. A white, triangular tent, covered at both ends so I can't see inside, is in an open area. I hear a small boy's laughter coming from inside the tent. Long, multicolored sashes, tied together and forming a multicolored snakelike pattern, are being pulled into the tent through a sphincter-like hole at one end. Suddenly, seated next to me, appears an East Indian Sage, about forty to fifty years old, with a radiant face. He, too, is laughing. He is dressed in orange saffron robes, which he wears comfortably and casually. He has

a graying beard. The Sage informs me that I need a teacher to help guide me into my next initiation. He suggests that I go to the bookstore and see what strikes me as interesting.

He then tells me to lie down on my stomach. He places one hand on the back of my head and the other on the lower end of my spine. I suddenly feel a current of energy, as though I were plugged into an electrical outlet. I begin to cry tears of appreciation. The Sage tells me he is healing my body... and I awaken.

In this dream the Sage tells Brugh Joy that he needs a teacher to guide him toward his next initiation. The dream culminates with an intimation of the Breakthrough experience that is possible on the path.

When the Time is Right

WE LIVE IN A TIME when unprecedented numbers of people are living to experience aging. Yet our culture lacks institutions to give guidance for those in the stage of the Search. Fortunately, efforts are underway to develop new institutions appropriate to our time and to the opportunity for initiation into Elderhood. Sage-ing® International, inspired by Reb Zalman Schachter-Shalomi, is one example of such an opportunity for those seeking a path toward *conscious aging*. Ron Pevny, the founder of the Center for Conscious Eldering and himself a practitioner of sage-ing, says he did not come to this work without going through his own Struggle, as shown in this dream he experienced when he entered midlife:

I am in my relatives' home in Durango, Colorado. It is my birthday. There is a card table set up and covered with wrapped gifts, which are for me. In my eagerness, I rush up to the table and accidentally knock against it. One of the gifts falls to the floor, and the wrapping partially opens. I see that it is a beautiful agate ring or pendant or bracelet or the like. I know that this is representative of the beautiful gifts on the table, and that I am not supposed to open these gifts yet. I feel bad for having crashed into the table. I awaken with the words, "All this will be yours when the time is right."

Ron Pevny notes that this dream came on his first vision quest training. His life at the time was filled with doubt and "dark nights," reflected in that Struggle: "I felt very flawed, stuck spiritually, and questioning whether these struggles would ever end. Finally, on the last night of the quest, when I was trying to stay awake all night, I just gave up struggling. It seemed nothing of consequence had happened on my quest, but I could no longer continue to work at making something happen. I let my eyes close, and was blessed with this dream which 30 years later is still alive in me and has helped me persist and stay on my path through many dark times since."

No Regrets

EVENTUALLY, "WHEN THE TIME IS RIGHT," more than 25 years later, Ron would have a powerful dream of the Return, which gave him the direction he needed to establish his program of wilderness vision quests, the signature program of the Center for Conscious Eldering:

> An important mystery play is happening, and I have been chosen to represent human beings on their deathbeds in this powerful ceremony. I am not dying myself, but am experiencing the dynamics of being about to die and learning what is necessary to die a good, peaceful death, free of baggage and emotional encumbrances.
>
> The ceremony has me being carried on a bier by several people. The only light is provided by torches and candles. The setting is one of great spiritual power and sacredness. I am carried to several stations where I experience specific teachings. One of these is a station where I am to make amends for anyone I have hurt in my life. I realize that I don't have many such amends to make. Neither this nor the other stations (which I don't remember as I write this) has a big impact on me in the dream.
>
> Then we come to the final station. Here tremendous power becomes focused, the heavens seem to open up, and I am deeply shaken as I hear the words, "No regrets. You can have no regrets. You must teach no regrets."
>
> I awaken with these words vibrating throughout my being. I go to the bathroom still feeling enveloped in this dream with these words repeating in my head. I go back to bed and I'm back in the dream, with me trying to understand how I am supposed to teach "no regrets." It seems this goes on for ages. Then, the scene shifts and I am with my rite-of-passage mentors from 30 years ago, Steven Foster and Meredith Little. They are teaching

a large group who listen with rapt attention in an outdoor amphitheater. Then, when they are finished, they tell me that it is now my turn to teach "no regrets." I try, but most of the people are leaving, the shape and acoustics of the setting change, and I find myself yelling just to be heard by a few people. Then Steven and Meredith tell me that before I can effectively teach "no regrets" I have to first truly understand and embody "no regrets" in my life. Then people will listen and no yelling will be necessary.

Ron Pevny commented about his dream: "This is perhaps the most powerful, impactful dream I have ever had. It has been pivotal in helping deepen my experiential and conceptual understanding of the inner work of conscious aging. It has given me a feeling of mandate for doing the work I am doing in the conscious aging movement. The inner work of transforming regret that helps people to die in peace and to enter the next life without negative karma — that is the same work that is necessary for dying to one's previous self-identifications, those encumbrances that prevent us from moving into the life stage of elder free of our old baggage, attachments, and other energy drainers. Those who shine most brightly as elders live with 'no regrets.'"

Changing the Culture — Slowly

NOTE THAT MORE THAN A QUARTER of a century elapsed between Ron Pevny's early vision quest dream and his dream of "No Regrets" which pointed him toward the practice that has become his distinctive contribution. The work of conscious eldering, as exemplified in Sage-ing® International, Second Journey, and other groups established in recent years, is not something that can be accomplished quickly. That fact seems to me all the more reason we commit our energies anew to the task of changing the culture.

Of late, I have been exploring how to live an integral life, how to access all the ages and stages of a life: the Spring student, the Summer Householder, the Autumn Forest Dweller, and the Winter Sage. And I have returned, like these seasons, again and again to Helen M. Luke's slim volume *Old Age* (New York: Parabola Books, 1987). Here, Helen Luke touches on *The Odyssey*, *King Lear*, *The Tempest*, and "Little Gidding." And she closes with an essay on Suffering.

When such gifts are given, something vibrates again — like a single note from a great harp, like the clear sound of a true word.

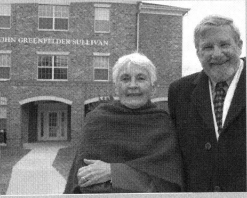

John Sullivan with his wife, Gregg, in front of the building at Elon University which was recently named in his honor.

A much-loved teacher at Elon University in North Carolina, Second Journey's "philosopher in residence" **John G. Sullivan** was named Elon's first Distinguished University Professor in 2002. His essays appear regularly in *Itineraries*, the Second Journey quarterly, and may be viewed online at SecondJourney.org/John'sCorner. He is the author of *The Spiral of the Seasons: Welcoming the Gifts of Later Life* (2009) and *The Fourfold Path to Wholeness: A Compass for the Heart* (2010), which are published by Second Journey. John is the author of two other books, *Living Large: Transformative Work at the Intersection of Ethics and Spirituality* and *To Come to Life More Fully: An East West Journey*.

Markers in the Stream

by John G. Sullivan

> *I would love to live / Like a river flows,*
> *Carried by the surprise / Of its own unfolding.*[1]

IMAGINE THE LONG ARC OF A LIFE, like a stream, flowing to the sea. Then think of markers in the stream. Some are universal or nearly so — a sequence of unfolding, a set of themes present throughout. Others are specific to this or that life. Each event challenges us. How will we respond? What will we learn? Who will we take ourselves to be? What will the Web of Life receive from our deepening?

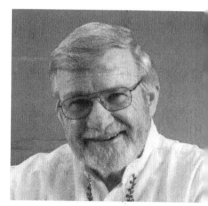

Here, we shall look at both the longer line of a lifetime and at some key transitions. In particular, I want to explore two initiations: the first into adulthood, the second into elderhood. Here is a verse to introduce the themes:

> One is the lifetime in which we now dwell.
> Two are the halves of life, upward and down.
> Four are the stages, a season for each.
> Two rites for entering each half of life.
> One is the Source and Goal, drawing our love.

From Half to Whole

Storyteller Michael Meade shares this fragment of a story:

> Once upon a time, in a village in Borneo, a Half-boy is born, a boy with only the right half of his body. He becomes a source of irritation, embarrassment, and confusion to himself, his family, and the entire village. Nonetheless, he grows and eventually reaches the age of adolescence. His halfness and incompleteness become unbearable to him and all around him. One day he leaves the village dragging himself along until he reaches a place where the road crosses a river. At that crossroad, he meets another youth who exists as only the left side, the other half of a person. They move towards each other as if destined to join. Surprisingly, when they reach each other, they begin to fight and roll in the dust. Then

they fall into the river. After a time, from the river there arises an entire youth with sides put together. The new youth walks toward a new village. He sees an old man and asks: "Can you tell me where I am? I have been struggling and don't know where I have arrived at." The old man says: "You have arrived home. You are back in the village where you were born. Now that you have returned whole, everyone can begin to dance and celebrate." And so it was and so it is.[2]

Perhaps today, two groups find themselves as Half-people. Springtime youth are entering the Arc of Ascent, seeking passage into the stage of adult Householder. Those facing retirement are entering the Arc of Descent, seeking passage into elderhood (i.e., into the stages of Autumn Forest Dweller and Winter Sage).[3]

As in the story, these two Half-people — youth and elders — seem destined for one another. How can youth be initiated if there are no elders to instruct them, if there are no elders to welcome them as they find the gifts they bring for the wider tribe? How can the young be seen and appreciated if there are no elders to dance with them and celebrate them? And how can those entering the second half of their lives (or final third)[4] find ways to develop and give their gifts if they are set apart and exiled from the next generation? Is it any wonder that the uninitiated old fight with the uninitiated young?

Yet perhaps there is even more to the story. Think of one of the Half persons as "First-Half-of-Life Person" (Youth-Householder). Think of the other Half person as "Second-Half-of-Life Person" (Forest Dweller-Sage). First and second half of life meet and engage in a struggle. They fall into a river and emerge whole. Now there is healing of four stages, and a new image emerges from the water: an integral person not fixed in any age but having access to all ages, access to all four capacities of life: (a) the experience and discovery of the Spring Student, (b) the experience and responsibilities of the Summer Householder, (c) the reintegration into the natural world of Autumn Forest Dweller, and (d) the light and easy dwelling in the ocean resources of Winter Sage. When we have access to this fourfold, then we are whole, then we are home in an integral way.

Four Themes Always Present, Ever Changing

ALL THAT UNFOLDS THROUGHOUT the lifetime is contained in seed at every moment. What are these seeds that need to be watered and tended throughout? I would say: (1) the soul-centric, (2) the communal-centric, (3) the nature or eco-centric, and (4) the cosmic- or spirit-centric.[5]

First, development throughout must be soul-centered. By soul I am pointing to the concrete and specific, the very particular perspectives, gifts, and contributions of each unique person. Frederick Buechner teaches us that to find our calling is "to find the interPart between our own deep gladness and the world's deep hunger."[6] Such is our soul work. Ultimately it is to be more and more our unique selves, our "perfectly imperfect" selves.

Second, development *must* be communal-centered throughout, seeing ourselves dwelling in a web of relationships ever expanding. We pass from child to adolescent and then to adult householder. As we do, our sense of community expands — family to peer group and then, through relationships of intimacy, into marriage and a new family. Beyond family, the circle expands to organizations and the larger communities in which they dwell. Under special conditions, we glimpse a circle expanding beyond tribe and nation to the whole human family. "I am a human being," says the playwright Terrence, "and nothing human is alien to me."

Third, development must be Earth-centered or eco-centric throughout. We are embedded in the natural world and interconnected with people, other animals, plants, and minerals — all of whom co-create and sustain our ecosystems. Seeds of this need to be tended at each stage.

Fourth, development must be cosmic-centered or spirit-centered throughout. We are developing in an unfolding universe and need a cosmology, a way of placing ourselves in the widest context so that we learn how to care for the whole and to align with the deep currents of what is unfolding. In this usage, "soul" points to what is most concrete and unique in us; "spirit" points to what is as vast as the universe and open to the Great Mystery that is within and beyond all that is.

Each of these seeds is watered by daily practice — the work of "coming to life more fully so as to serve life more wisely and more nobly."[7] Each of these seeds is linked with a stage.

- Youth are drawn into soul work, finding and developing their gifts.
- Householders care for the human community, ever widening its scope.
- Forest Dwellers (early elders) expand the circle to include all species: people, other animals, plants and minerals, plus

ecosystems such as mountains and meadows, rivers and oceans, forests and plains.
- Winter Sages (later elders) expand the family still further, returning to the place where Source, Self, and Circle of All Life meet. Paradoxically, Winter Sages are aware of both the vastest of horizons and the most intimate of practices, namely dwelling in "present moment, wonderful moment."[8]

As noted, in the midst of this stage sequence, we experience marker events. Some are relatively universal. Think of birth, puberty, first love, first sexual experience, marriage, childbirth, the end of childbearing, the end of full-time work, the rediscovery of nature, and finally a confrontation with death.[9] Other markers are less predictable: accidents and sickness, injustices suffered, hurt inflicted, reversals at work, the death or injury of loved ones, and on and on. Through it all, we are called to daily practices of stillness and service — quiet inward deepening for the sake of serving; outward serving for the sake of deepening all our kin.[10]

On the Arc of Ascent, the daily work of Spring Students and Summer Householders is dominated by a kind of striving: striving to actualize an ideal of who we might be, could be, should be, striving to maximize our potential. The beauty here is that we are striving for excellence, desiring to be open to more and ever more. We are learning to care for units larger than ourselves. Our striving is not for ourselves only. Still, in this striving — even for good things — a trap appears: a kind of perfectionism. Under its spell, we are like the greyhounds in a race, chasing a mechanical rabbit that stays always beyond our reach. So we are ever falling short of who we think we are meant to be. Striving, striving, striving. Then comes a turning, and we enter the Arc of Descent. Down into Autumn release and further down into Winter waters.

What signals this reversal? Perhaps we step down from the work we have done as a career. We retire from the tasks that have shaped us. We release from being so defined by roles and beliefs. We surrender into a greater unknown. Our children are grown; grandchildren arrive. For women, menopause arrives, and they know in a bodily way that the years of potential childbearing have come to an end. Both men and women enter, in different ways, the Arc of Descent through Autumn into Winter. The waterfall energy is moving downward and inward. We can resist, or we can align with the energy. In Autumn, we can return to a new appreciation of our place in the natural world. In the starkness of

Winter, we can release still further, returning to the moment, to the here and now — a here and now in which everything is contained. In the Arc of Descent, we let go of striving to change the world, let go of seeking to control others, let go of achieving some ideal or other for ourselves. We let go of thinking life is about us at all! We become a window allowing the whole to be present in and through us from a unique place, a unique history of choices.[11]

The fourfold is indeed an image of wholeness: four directions, four seasons, four stages of life.[12] Perhaps we can hold out a new image of the human by not imagining ourselves at a particular age, but instead by bringing together the capacities of all four ages: Spring Student, Summer Householder, Autumn Forest Dweller, and Winter Sage. Let us consider again this possibility. Then becoming fully human would mean being:

- Ever young, ever learning, ever returning to "beginner's mind."
- Ever in Householder service to those given to our care, as we expand the circle to the full human family.
- Ever in Forest Dweller mode, releasing, turning, and returning to the natural world, experiencing interconnection with the Circle of all Life, the Great Family.
- Ever in the joyous sagely way of "loving what is,"[13] ever reflecting more fully the place where the three worlds touch: Self, Source, and the Circle of All Life.

A beautiful image of harmony. Four stages coming together for the sake of all beings.

Growing Up: the Initiation of Fire:
From Spring Student to Summer Householder

IN THE EARLY 1900S, ANTHROPOLOGIST Arnold van Gennep distinguished three phases in a rite of passage ceremony, namely (a) severance, (b) threshold, and (c) incorporation.[14]

Before the beginning of the rite, the elders prepare the initiates, instructing them as to what will happen and its meaning. The elder men prepare the adolescent boys. The elder women prepare the adolescent girls. The stage is set to hear what it means to be a man, what it means to be a woman, how to be with the mysteries of sexuality and spirituality as understood by the tribe in the widest and deepest way, how to find one's gifts and serve the community. Think here of a Native American vision quest, a process that is being revived by much wilderness work.[15]

The Severance Phase — In this phase, the initiates may be sent into the wilderness to fast and "cry for a vision."[16] Severance marks an ending — and with it, some grieving for what was, some fear of what will be, some gratefulness at shedding an old stage, some excitement at entering a new.

The Threshold Phase — In the midst of the experience, the initiates are in a "between state." Brought face to face with powers in the natural world far greater than themselves, they undergo trial and hardship. They are instructed to be open to the living and the dead. Open to all manifestations of the Great Family: humans, animals, plants, and minerals. All is spirit-infused, including places such as lakes and mountains, trees, rock formations, open meadows. The initiates confront deep fear. By fasting and other prayerful practices they open to altered states of awareness. They dream dreams and see visions. They undergo a symbolic death and rebirth. In all this, they seek their destiny, their particular way of serving the community, their uniqueness-become-gift. They are being changed in ways they can hardly understand. Fearful and fascinating are the mysteries.

The Phase of Incorporation — Here, the initiates are welcomed back into the community, with a new status and sometimes a new name. Each youth recounts his or her experience, and the elders help interpret and confirm the change. All this is not for the individual alone. It is for the sake of the tribe continuing. Now the young boy is a man; the young girl, a woman. They assume new tasks not for themselves alone. (They serve the tribe.) They assume new tasks not by themselves alone. (They are companioned in their service.) They assume new tasks not by their own powers alone. (They participate in the Great Mystery and draw strength from powers greater than themselves.)

Growing Down: the Second Initiation —
From Householder to Forest Dweller/Sage

CARL JUNG SPEAKS ABOUT a second initiation, calling it "The Night Sea Journey." I think of it as going over the waterfall and descending like a drop of water moving ever deeper into the great sea. The Arc of Descent has begun. Less a matter of doing, more a matter of *not* doing, A matter of following the Watercourse Way,[17] using its own gravitational arc. Receiving. Releasing. Returning. Remembering. Coming back to what was and is and ever shall be.

What might that second initiation look like if we partly rediscovered it, partly reinvented it, for our times? What would it be to mark the Arc of Descent with its own initiation? Here is a possible template, using the three phases already described.[18]

Preparation[19] — In the spirit of Forest Dweller and Sage, preparation calls us to a work in our time. Joanna Macy calls this work "The Great Turning," taking us from an industrial growth society to a life-sustaining society. Thomas Berry calls this "The Great Work."[20] This work beckons us to step into a new cosmology, a new universe story large enough for science, art, and spirituality.

Suppose we invoke — in space — the Great Family: the spirits of all the creatures of Earth and sky and sea; all the elements — earth, water, fire, and air; and the Great Mystery that breathes through all.

Suppose we invoke — in time — the beings of the three times, our ancestors (human and all the other species), our contemporaries (human and all the other species), and all the children yet-to-be-born (of all species).

Suppose further that we open to a context greater still — one that adds to everything so far invoked — the place where the three worlds meet. The place where Source, deep Self, and the Circle of All Life intersect. Suppose we also ask a blessing from the Mysterious Source that sustains us and flows through all things; ask a blessing from our own deep self; ask a blessing from the depth dimension in all things.

The Severance Phase — During this phase when we leave one way of being and acclimate to another, the initiates into elderhood may enter the wilderness literally or invoke this wilderness context in other ways. Surely, it is in the spirit of Forest Dweller to find the Great Mystery in all of life and in each place. Surely, our awareness of the greater powers is heightened as we fast and pray and cry for a vision for the remainder of our life. Surely, we will enter the great silence, the solitude and solidarity of contemplative openness, the simplicity and humility of our fragile self.

The Threshold Phase — In this phase, which is the experience itself, we are falling like the leaves, falling like the drop going over the waterfall on its way to the sea. The way is letting go and letting be. Relinquishing control. Loving what is. Learning to live until our death and to die again and again to our illusions and misdirected fantasies. We are all the characters in the drama, the heroes and villains, the major players and those who appear for only a moment. And we need the help of the universe. As Rumi says:

> Pale sunlight,
> Pale the wall.
>
> Love moves away.
> The light changes.
>
> I need more grace
> than I thought.[21]

Perhaps we review our life, acknowledging what we have done and failed to do. We enter forgiveness work by bringing to mind those we have hurt and those who have hurt us.[22] We bring to light in gentle ways the bright and dark shadows[23] of our youth and Householder, of our Forest Dweller and Sage as these shadows are manifesting right here and now. We are supported in this by all whom we have invoked. What are our gifts at this stage? What is the place where our deep gladness and the world's deep hunger touch? Where is the place where our hearts open to all of life? How will we continue to access the youthful Student-in-us, the adult Householder-in-us, the elder Forest-Dweller-in-us, and the timeless Sage-in-us? We are dying to a way of being that sought to accomplish and to control ourselves and others, sought to bring our answers to the world. Now we learn to shift to asking questions and listening to what each moment brings to teach us. We have died to one way of seeing and being. We are symbolically reborn into another way. We are beginners at this new possibility. And we have all we need and all we seek.

The Phase of Incorporation —
Gifts for the larger community

IMAGINE MEETING WITH FELLOW ELDERS in a council setting to clarify the meaning of what each newly welcomed elder brings. Perhaps such meetings take place periodically — in a retreat setting conducive to stillness and service. Let them provide a context to explore personal deepening and community enrichment, a context combining the particularity of soul work and the vastness of spirit dwelling.[24]

To close, let us call to mind and heart these words from the poet and playwright, Christopher Fry:[25]

> Thank God our time is now when wrong
> Comes up to face us everywhere,
> Never to leave us till we take
> The longest stride of soul we ever took.
> Affairs are now soul size.
> The enterprise
> Is exploration into God. . . .
> It takes
> So many thousand years to wake,
> But will you wake for pity's sake!

In *Active Hope: How to Face the Mess We're in Without Going Crazy*, renowned Earth elder Joanna Macy and her colleague Chris Johnstone offer the essential guidebook for everyone awakening to both the perils and potentials of our planetary moment. Joanna has long exemplified what it means to live a life of spiritual activism and courageous compassion. Now, in this clearly written and compelling manual of cultural transformation, she guides us to find hope where we might least have thought to look — within our own hearts and souls, and in our interdependence with all life — and then to boldly act on that hope as visionary artisans of life-enhancing cultures. *Active Hope* amply delivers on the promise of its subtitle. To the future beings of the twenty-second century, this book might turn out to be the most important of the twenty-first.

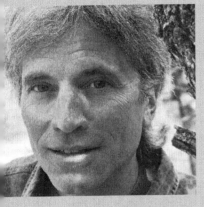

Bill Plotkin

Bill Plotkin, founder of Colorado's Animas Valley Institute, is a depth psychologist, wilderness guide, and agent of cultural transformation. Author of *Soulcraft: Crossing into the Mysteries of Nature and Psyche* (an experiential guidebook) and *Nature and the Human Soul: Cultivating Wholeness and Community in a Fragmented World* (a nature-based stage model of human development through the entire lifespan), he has guided thousands of people through nature-based initiatory passages in the underworld of soul, including a contemporary, Western adaptation of the pan-cultural vision quest.

Invitations to Practice

Releasing the Past
by Ron Pevny

The journey into a conscious elderhood is one that very much involves recognizing and dealing with both dying and living, ending and beginning. In the journey we recognize that these powerful dynamics are intimately woven together, as we concurrently prepare for two endings and two beginnings. Both physical death and the passage into conscious elderhood are, for the psyche, a death to an old way of being. And they are both doorways into new chapters in life's journey of growth.

One of the core tenets of conscious or spiritual eldering (two names for the same transformative inner work) is that the work that prepares us to be at peace as we leave this life is the same work that prepares us to become conscious elders. It involves healing our past and leaving behind our self-identification with our previous life stage. Once done, we can move without encumbrance into the mysterious next chapter that awaits us.

Whenever we reflect on our mortality, death, and what may follow, most everyone hopes to die in peace. We want to be able to feel that our lives have been well lived, that we have done our best to use our gifts, that we have loved and been loved, and that we can let go of this life with grace and without regret. In her poem, "When Death Comes," the poet Mary Oliver, captures this desire exquisitely:

> When it's over, I don't want to wonder
> if I have made of my life something particular, and real.
> I don't want to find myself sighing and frightened,
> or full of argument.
> I don't want to end up simply having visited this world.[1]

Yet, many people do not die "frightened or full of argument." Colleagues, friends, and participants in our Choosing Conscious Elderhood retreats who work with hospice all say that those who die the most peaceful deaths are those who come to their deathbeds unburdened by a lifetime's accumulation of resentments, regrets, dysfunctional relationships, unhealed grief, and closed hearts. Besides manifesting as emotional turmoil, such unfinished business often results in prolonged physical agony while the dying person clings to a life that feels incomplete and unfulfilled. Often the greatest gift that hospice spiritual directors give to those in their charge is help dealing with unfinished business so that the patients can let go of this life with hearts that are more open to love and peace.

A practice called The Death Lodge draws upon powerful imagery to bring together various aspects of the inner work of healing the past. Because the work of this practice feels so very freeing and enlivening, some of our retreat participants prefer to also call it *The Life Lodge*. Choose whatever name you prefer.

The Death Lodge Tradition

I first learned about the Death Lodge many years ago from my teachers Steven Foster and Meredith Little, the pioneers in the modern rite-of-passage movement. Their book on vision questing, *The Roaring of the Sacred River*, describes the Death Lodge as "a little house away from the village where people go when they want to tell everyone they are ready to die."[2] Foster and Little attribute the Death Lodge concept to the Cheyenne tribe of the Native Americans of the Plains. To begin to understand the power of this practice, imagine you are an indigenous person who has grown old and weary of this life and knows your death is near. You attend to those practical matters that need to be done at the end of your life such as passing on your belongings. Then you leave village life behind to enter a special place, the Death Lodge, where you will focus on reviewing your life, repairing or completing your relationships, and preparing to move from this life into the mystery beyond.

In the Death Lodge you remember the important events, dynamics, and people of your life. Situations may look very different from the perspective of your approaching death than they did at the time they happened. You reflect on how you have used your gifts. You acknowledge your strengths and weaknesses, and forgive yourself for the harm you have done to others. You explore your relationship with the Great

Spirit, throughout your life and now particularly at this point of nearing your passage into the great unknown. Then, when the time feels right, you invite those in your village who have played important roles in your life to come visit you, one at a time. This is the time for bringing your relationships to completion. You and each of your visitors do whatever needs to be done so that your relationship feels complete, with no unfinished business. Now, with death approaching, the dynamics of these relationships may appear quite different than previously. You thank and honor each other for the role you have played in each other's lives, and you say goodbye. Once this work is complete, you are at peace with your life, your community, and your God and are ready to move into the world of spirit.

The Death Lodge Practice As a Rite of Passage

We obviously live in a very different world than the indigenous societies where the death that happens at life's major passages is acknowledged and honored as part of the cycle of life and is consciously prepared for. Our modern world has few, if any, true rites of passage that require a conscious death to our old sense of self as a prerequisite for moving into life's next stage. However, deep inside each of us is an indigenous self that remembers that nature's cycles of life and death, with death being necessary for new life, are also the cycles of our lives. Conscious eldering is very much a process of becoming conscious of these rhythms as they operate in us, making way for the birth of new possibility when we begin to leave midlife adulthood. I believe that one reason the Death Lodge practice resonates so deeply with our retreat participants is that its imagery taps into that wisdom in us that knows about how to align ourselves with the cycle of life and death.

The following is my recommendation for how you can employ the Death Lodge as work to support your passage into a conscious elderhood. By doing so, you will also keep your inner work up to date as you draw ever nearer to life's final passage. First, be aware that Death Lodge work is not something you do one time and then it's complete. It is best viewed as a practice that you periodically revisit as part of your commitment to your inner growth. I encourage you to view Death Lodge work as a sacred ritual done with care and intention. If possible, do it outside in a natural place that will help align you with nature's cycles. Give yourself enough time to do focused inner work without distraction. Ideally, find a small area that has the feel of an enclosed little house or lodge, such as a spot in a grove of trees or a cave-like space amid rocks or under overhanging bushes,

Before you enter, offer a prayer or state an intention that the sacred, however you name it, be with you supporting and guiding your work. You might bless and purify your Lodge with incense or bring in some flowers. Be sure to bring along your journal and perhaps an object that you consider sacred. This work is most profound if you approach it imagining, as best you can, that you have only a few weeks left to live and that you are indeed preparing to die. You never know. That may indeed be the case.

Once inside your Death Lodge, be quiet and wait to see what type of life-completion/life-healing work feels most alive for you. Are you aware of a painful experience that needs to be examined, felt more deeply, and reframed so you can understand how it contributed previously, or can now contribute, to your growth? Are there regrets that disempower you and diminish your sense of self-worth and the worth of your life? If so, how can you change the way you relate to these regrets? Are there experiences of joy or accomplishment you want to spend time reliving — and perhaps reviewing as a way to remember your strengths and gifts? What is the state of your relationship with the Spirit (however you name it) that is your source and essence? You might want to spend time focused on gratitude for all of the incredible journey that is your life.

For many people, the most important work of the Death Lodge involves bringing healing and completion to relationships. In your Lodge you have the opportunity to spend time, in spirit, with people who have been significant in your life. What needs to be said to bring completion and, if needed, healing to each particular relationship? What need is there to forgive, and are you willing to do so? What contribution has the other made to your life and growth that needs to be acknowledged? How can you best honor the other before you say goodbye?

Who to Invite for Relationship Completion

There are several different possibilities for who you can invite into your Death Lodge (and sometimes you may find someone knocking at the door without an invitation — a clear indication that they belong there).

- You can become aware of others who are alive, with whom healing needs to happen, and with whom a face-to-face conversation is possible if you make the effort. You can use the Death Lodge to practice what you will say to them and to make the commitment to try your best to meet with them in person.
- You can invite others who are alive but with whom a face-to-face meeting is an impossibility for whatever reasons. Picture them in your Lodge with you and imagine yourself talking to their spirits — to the best in them — saying what you need to say and hearing their response. Using your journal for such conversations can help make this process more tangible. The Gestalt process of moving back and forth from one seat to another is also helpful for some people.
- You can invite people who have died with whom you have never had or you missed the opportunity to share what's in your heart. Does grief need to be expressed? Anger? Gratitude? Forgiveness? A request for forgiveness? Again, speak to their spirit and imagine what that wise, loving essence in them has to say to you. If you cannot connect with a sense of what their spirit has to say, only remembering their personality selves which may have been hurtful to you, that's OK. Speak the truth of your heart, doing your best to recognize and honor their role in your growth while acknowledging the pain they may have caused you.
- For many people, the most important and difficult Death Lodge work is the work of forgiving and honoring themselves — or, to be more precise, those parts of themselves that have made errors and poor decisions, have hurt others, are weak, are imperfect. Nothing is more disempowering — closing our hearts and filling us with conflict — than self-loathing. Here we have the opportunity to forgive these parts of ourselves for their weakness and to thank them for what they have taught

us about our shadows and our values. From the perspective of our conscious and aware selves we can dialogue with and extend love to these parts of us (using our journal can be very helpful) with the goal of reintegrating disowned aspects of ourselves. The more we do so, the more whole we become.

A Retreat Participant's Healing Experience

I have been privileged to hear from retreat participants many stories about their use of the Death Lodge, on retreat and as a regular practice in their lives. I'd like to close by sharing the deeply transformative Death Lodge experience of Annette, as related in her own words.

> There was a moment in time that excruciatingly split my life into the "before" and "after" — a recalibration of time that set that moment as the moment relative to which all prior and subsequent events are now remembered. The zero on my X-axis of time: June 17, 1999.
>
> The phone rang. A voice said, "Molly has shot herself." She had been at her father's house. In a blur of events I found myself at the emergency room hearing a physician say the words. She is dead. She was 15. My daughter was brilliant, beautiful, happy, precious, and so very loved by so many people. So loved by me. A moment of drama over a boy, an argument with her father, an available loaded pistol, and she gave up every sweetly anticipated experience of growing into adulthood on this earth.
>
> My son, my living daughter, and I lived in a stunned and painful silence, patient and tolerant of each other's process in grief, absorbing our new reality. A woman from the funeral home brought me a small velvet bag with Molly's jewelry: a watch that I had bought her, a silver butterfly pendant on a chain (the symbol of her closest girlfriends), and silver earrings. She had worn these when she died. The velvet bag held these precious objects. I held it for many months.
>
> Four years later, around Thanksgiving, I began to feel human, and my son and I remarked that we were smiling.
>
> Twelve years later, a colleague sent me a link to a retreat on conscious eldering, to be held at a small retreat center near Mt. Shasta. I was put

off by the rude suggestion that I might be aging and that I might need to deal with it in a thoughtful way — a clear sign that I needed to go. We were to bring to the retreat significant objects from our lives to create an altar, objects that we felt identified us in some way. The thought of Molly, ever present, kept a lump in my throat and the sorrow just slightly beneath the surface. Suicide is different from any other death. There is a stigma. It is impossible to explain, but only other parents of children who have taken their own lives seem to understand the complexity. I took a photo of Molly.

My conscious eldering cohorts were loving, gentle, and experienced in a variety of ways, each bringing a rich perspective to life and life's cycle. I was prepared for my day of solitude and fasting on the mountain, and content as I approached my little sanctuary of solitude. The snow had melted enough to leave patches of dry earth, on which grew burgeoning wild grasses and plants pushing their way to the sun. I sprawled on my back to watch the clouds and feel the mountain. It felt safe. It was beautiful. I spoke to a bee. I explored. I came across a circle of stones that had been laid around a small pit, an indention in the earth as if scooped out to form a bowl. This place, previously created for some sacred moment in another's life, became my Death Lodge. Shasta offered the perfect blending of death and renewal. Felled trees, rotting where they landed, created swells in the landscape, changing the flow of run-off, adjusting the topography, forever changing the landscape by their death. How perfect. The beauty and symmetry of life amidst decomposition prepared me for my Death Lodge work.

It felt odd, speaking aloud to my deceased family members — grandparents, aunts and uncles, and friends who were so dear. There were many with whom I shared this moment, saving Molly for last. I spoke to my friend, Ann, who had promised as she lay dying that she would find Molly and let me know, if there was any way possible, that she was okay. In my Death Lodge I loved talking to Ann about what she had meant to me in life and in death.

Then came my friend Bob, who had shared his death from pancreatic cancer with me just nine months before. His friendship was transforming. A few months before his death, I had been seated next to him in a pew at 18-year-old Brian's memorial service, with the strange understanding that his service would be next. Bob's remarks had been profound: "How perfect. Brian was in a perfect place in his life. Why do we get hung up in the idea that more is better?"

Bob's death a few months later was intimate and tender, filled with grace and love, as he denied fear with the words, "Why would I be afraid when I get to fall asleep, relieved of pain, and awaken staring into the eyes of my God?" I spoke to Bob in my Death Lodge. I thanked him for taking me with him down that path of transforming fear, as far as I could go. He gave me, in his death, the ability to see life more clearly. All those who were present for me in my Death Lodge had all felt receptive to my gratitude and amends. Now I was ready to speak to Molly.

For the first time in 12 years, I felt her presence. I spoke to her, and then with her, about my love for her, my horror at her death, and my struggle with the permanence of her choice. I wanted, yearned, for her to have lived out her life — to have survived that painful moment and to experience all that life has to offer — and to find the peace and joy that come from maturity and self-acceptance. I wanted just once more to hear the sound of her voice. I wanted her as the receptacle for immense love and devotion that had welled in my heart with no place to go for so many years. I asked forgiveness, for what I do not know. I told her that if I had hurt her, I no longer remembered having done so and wanted her to know that I had to quit trying to figure it out. She understood. I then heard Bob's words: "Why do we dwell on the thought that more is better?" Indeed. I had lived for 15 years with this precious, clever, beautiful, spontaneous, loving child in delight and yet spent almost all of the following 12 years in pain over her death rather than in awe of her life and the gift of her creation in my body and birth into my family. I felt the weight lift in an instant. Tears rolling down my cheek, I pledged to honor her by living in gratitude for her life rather than in misery over her death.

Then, a butterfly appeared from the trees and fluttered through the death lodge, encircling my head and gracing me with its beauty. As she flew away, I said, "No, come back!" and then caught myself in a smile, chuckling at my own compulsion to want more. From that day, I have loved Molly in joy more than sorrow. My tears are now of gratitude. I miss her terribly. I am so fortunate to have had her in my life.

Resources
Contributors
Notes

Endings and Intimations

Snow trickles away on gray ground
a cold sun sinks sullen in western sky,
as flowers fade, leaves turn and clocks demand endings.
Will our bright children come to a good or bad end?
In the hall, the curtain falls and applause drifts off
after the aging player struts boldly and bows
near the stage edge to delay the certain change of
his final fall into who knows.
Is there a clue beyond passing and more passing?
Perhaps in every breath finishing with a still point, an eternal moment
like the nano-pause between raised baton and ensuing sound,
in a microsecond of a real though fleeting stop,
so light, so quick, so there and gone,
as between our breathings we sense a dwelling presence
from beyond the race track of time
when we hear a blessed echo from an unknown cliff,
a quiet hymn of hope for every child even now.

— Eugene C. Bianchi[†]

[†] From *Ear to the Ground: Poems from the Long View* by Eugene C. Bianchi (Parson's Porch Publishers, 2013).

REFLECTIONS OF A LIFELONG READER

BY BARBARA KAMMERLOHR

*F**rom the moment I could read, books* and articles provided answers to many questions about life's mysteries. They were particularly helpful during early retirement years when I had no clear idea about how to negotiate the journey ahead. But books seemed to fail me as I worked to understand late-life spirituality, one of the most important concepts for acquiring the wisdom and tranquility that are hallmarks of a true elder.

An essential part of entrance into the metaphorical autumn and winter seasons of life is working with the emergence of this unique kind of spirituality. It is a fascinating topic, full of wonder and adventure as we undertake the journey to embrace this puzzling, sometimes mystical, stage of life. It is a topic that both intrigued and eluded me as the stirrings within my own soul cried for understanding, and the copious amount of literature on the topic piled up in my study. Nothing I read brought me to a deeper understanding of my soul.

Most of the books I have read since committing to aging consciously benefitted me greatly. Learning about the developmental tasks of the autumn years and interacting with people who were accomplishing those tasks successfully helped create a retirement in synch with my own personality — a great adventure. Unfortunately, the demands of late autumn/early winter are slightly different, and the demands of the soul for more recognition change one's perspective dramatically. In spite of my 35-year meditation practice and life-long pursuit of the elusive "spiritual," something had changed and cried for my attention.

I found plenty to read about late-life spirituality, but nothing captured the essence of the topic the way earlier books on conscious aging had done. It was as if I had acquired a lot of information, but missed the central point. Only after a decision to review all the books in my library — a task I never completed — did the awaited "aha!" moment come.

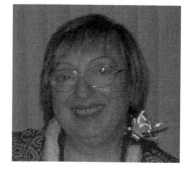

The wisdom behind that "aha" explained it all. Late-life spirituality is fundamentally unique for each of us — a journey in search of the transcendent, a journey deep into our own souls to discover, experience, and learn about the true self. Knowing one's own soul is a challenge for any author. There is no one who can teach me about this one soul. I can only learn by experiencing the journey inward.

Earlier, this self appeared sporadically as we expressed ourselves in choices of career, family, friendships, hobbies, and in the way we approached life's challenges, sometimes honestly, sometimes shrinking from the task. We now have the time to become acquainted with that soul — to reflect on how all of the parts — career, family, relationships, and aspirations — painted the picture of one unique soul. No more career ladders to climb. No more children to sit up with all night. No need to worry about getting the loan on the house or where to spend the limited number of vacation days. Moreover, reflection on the struggles of earlier years provides clues to understanding who we really are, where our soul has been trying to take us, and where it is going.

No book, or combination of books and articles, can teach me or you about late-life spirituality. This must be an experience to which our own souls lead us. The experience will be so unique that no one else can describe it. There is no "literature" that accurately describes this "cruise" — only a few publications that can point to milestones and give tips for a successful journey.

That disclaimer finished, however, there are books that contain fundamental concepts helpful to this journey. In reading, I did discover important concepts about late-life spirituality. The most important ones I share in the paragraphs below:

- There are two parts to our Earth journey: the outer journey which happens primarily during the first half of life, and the inner journey, a major developmental task of life's late afternoon.
- Institutions in our culture prepare and support citizens in the first part of the journey. Guidance counselors and career coaches help with career development. A variety of "experts" focus on accumulation of riches, how to get a job, how to keep a job, leadership skills, caring for a family, relationships, etc. However, most of us know little about the second part of the journey that takes us inward to our true selves. In fact, many are not aware of it, many do not undertake it, and too many fear it.

- Other cultures, especially in the East and traditional Native Americans, honor and support the inner work of aging. Elders are sought for their wisdom and supported by extended family. Scholars of ancient Rome and Greece point to vestiges of a western culture that once honored elderhood, but this aspect of western culture seemed to disappear with the destruction of Rome.
- For us, in 21st-century western culture, the inner journey must be consciously undertaken, even though deepening stirrings of desire for contact with the soul occur naturally as part of the aging process.
- There are a variety of techniques that help with this, but they must be chosen carefully and used regularly. Daily meditation is the one discipline recommended by most "experts" on aging. Other techniques that can be helpful include: journaling, dream work, awareness practices, artistic endeavors, forgiveness practices, visualization, yoga, tai chi, prayer, and therapeutic writing of all kinds. None of these are unique to conscious aging. Religious institutions, adult schools, senior centers, and philosophical organizations teach these practices to individuals of all ages who undertake the work of contacting their own souls on a deeper level.

While it was my own meditation practice that led me to the most satisfying understanding of late-life spirituality, the following books contained helpful information. The reader interested in the concepts of late-life spirituality will find them helpful — but not a substitute for the inner work that must be done.

Chittister, Joan. *The Gift of Years: Growing Older Gracefully*. BlueBridge, 2008.
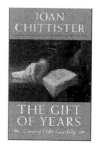
A compendium of inspiration and wisdom for people facing aging and for everyone who wants to live a spiritually centered life. The book has chapters on such topics as regret, meaning, fear, joy, newness, accomplishment, dreams, solitude, faith. Chittister said of her book, "This book is about the enterprise of embracing the blessings of this time and overcoming the burdens of it. That is the spiritual task of later life."

Erikson, Erik H. *The Life Cycle Completed* (Extended Version with New Chapters on the Ninth Stage of Development by Joan M. Erikson). Norton, 1997.

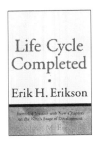

For decades, Erikson's concept of the stages of human development significantly influenced the field of contemporary psychology. However, his conceptualization of the ninth, and final, stage of life was missing until he, himself, entered that stage. The concepts in this book grew from Erikson's own inner journey and were published by his wife and coworker after his death. Both his insights and courage in articulating the experience of advanced old age give inspiration to those of us who are beginning this stage of our own journey.

Hillman, James. *The Force of Character and the Lasting Life*. Random House, 1999.

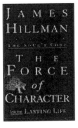

The Force of Character takes us on an enriching journey through the three states of aging: lasting, the deepening that comes with longevity; leaving, the preparation for departure; left, the special legacy we each bestow on our survivors. At the same time he is writing of these stages, Hillman explores the nature of character. "Character requires the additional years," he wrote. "The last years confirm and fulfill character. Far from blunting or dulling the self, the accumulation of experience concentrates the essence of our being, heightening our individual mystery and unique awareness of life."

Hollister, James. *Finding Meaning in the Second Half of Life: How to Finally, Really Grow Up*. Gotham Books, 2005.

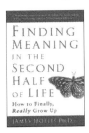

This book, written by a Jungian analyst, has become a classic and "must read" for anyone beginning the journey of conscious aging. However, it is the three final chapters that are relevant to those trying to understand late-life spirituality. These chapters are: "Recovering Mature Spirituality in a Material Age," "Swampland Visitations," and "The Healing of the Soul." Even those who read the book earlier in their journey will find these chapters particularly enlightening.

Rohr, Richard. *Falling Upward: A Spirituality for the Two Halves of Life*. Jossey-Bass, 2011.

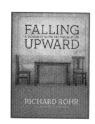

This book by Franciscan priest Richard Rohr is a map of the inner journey, detailing the differences between that journey during the first and second halves of life. The author proposed an alternative title, "Tips for the Road." Rohr contends that many people are not aware of the further journey during life's second half. Even fewer consciously undertake it. "We are given a span of years to discover our own soul, to choose it and to live our own destiny to the full. If we do not, our True Self will never be offered again."

Rumi: Paintings and Poems. Translated by Maryam Mafi and Azima Melita Kolin. Element Books, 2011.

A short collection of poems by Rumi translated into English. Full-color art work that also evokes the wonder of the great mystic serves as a stimulus for contemplation. Here is one example of his poetry for those who have not been introduced to the great Sufi master:

> You are searching the world for treasure
> but the real treasure is yourself.
> If you are tempted by bread
> you will find only bread.
> What you seek for you become.

Schachter-Shalomi, Zalman and Ronald S. Miller. *From Age-ing to Sage-ing: A Profound New Vision of Growing Older*. Grand Central Publishing, 1995.

This is the classic work that defined a vision for growing older with dignity and enthusiasm. Its author was the inspiration for Second Journey, Sage-ing® International, and other organizations that support visions of how to work with the gifts of age. Most readers who have undertaken the work of conscious aging have already read this and other works by this rabbi who freely uses experiences with his own aging process to help the rest of us understand the process unfolding within ourselves. However, it is worth reading a second time to focus on the implications for understanding late-life spirituality.

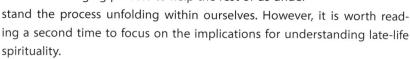

Sherman, Edmund. *Contemplative Aging: A Way of Being in Later Life*. Gordian Knot Books, 2010.

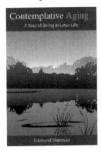

Written by a practicing gerontologist and retired university professor, this is the most comprehensive book on late-life spirituality I have read. It has everything: theoretical perspectives from the academic and clinical world, stories of the author's clients' journeys into the self, illustrations from the author's own personal search, and information about how to experience a more peaceful and aware way of being through contemplative practices.

Smith, Houston with Jeffrey Paine. *Tales of Wonder: Adventures Chasing the Divine, an Autobiography*. Harper-Collins, 2011.

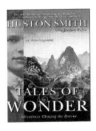

This is the latest autobiography by the 92-year-old scholar who wrote and published the definitive scholarly work on *The World's Religions*, the college professor who introduced us to the commonalities of all great religions. *Tales of Wonder*, however, is written from the nursing home in Berkeley, California, where he currently lives. It is a book from the heart, brief and humbly written, the perfect example of writing that integrates all of the various, conflicting aspects of a lifetime.

Sullivan, John G. *The Spiral of the Seasons: Welcoming the Gifts of Later Life*. Second Journey Publications, 2009.

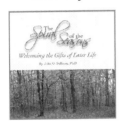

A short, inspirational, artistically rendered collection of four essays that overlay the four stages of life on the four seasons of the year. "In Spring, we are in the stage of the Student. In Summer, we move to the stage of the Householder. In Autumn, we enter the stage of the Forest Dweller. In Winter, we drop into the state of the Sage."

About the Contributors

Bolton Anthony, who founded Second Journey in 1999, has worked as a teacher of English and creative writing to undergraduates, and as a public librarian, university administrator, and social change activist. He lives with his wife, Lisa, in Chapel Hill, North Carolina. [pp. 5, 11, 59, 117, 171]

Robert C. Atchley, distinguished Professor of Gerontology Emeritus at Miami University, Ohio, where he directed the Scripps Gerontology Center, is the author of Social Forces and Aging and Aging and Spirituality. He lives in Lafayette, Colorado. [pp. 23, 153]

Karen A. Bannister is a writer and editor living in British Columbia, Canada with her family. She holds a Masters in Comparative Literature and the Arts. Her Web site is www.karenbannister.ca. [p. 93]

Jim Clark, a retired software developer with a love for cosmology, lives in Seattle, Washington. [p. 191]

Betsy Crites, MPH, co-founded and served as Director of Witness for Peace, a nationwide, faith-based organization committed to nonviolence in support of just U.S. policies in Latin America. She also served with Nonviolent Peaceforce accompanying human rights defenders in Guatemala, with Metta Center on Nonviolence as interim director, and as Director of N.C. Peace Action. She lives in Durham, North Carolina. [pp. 125, 167]

Judith Helburn, a Certified Sage-ing® Leader, is active in Sageing® International. She was one of two recipients of the first Reb Zalman Leadership Award in 2010. She works with several senior groups in Austin, Texas, has also been President of Story Circle Network, and leads a monthly writing circle. [p. 159]

Ellen S. Jaffe, a writer, teacher, and psychotherapist, is the author of *Writing Your Way: Creating a Personal Journal*, *Feast of Lights* (a novel for young adults), and two poetry collections, including the forthcoming *Skinny-Dipping with the Muse* (Guernica, 2014.) She lives in Hamilton, Ontario. www.ellen-s-jaffe.com. [p.109]

Barbara Kammerlohr, author and reviewer, is currently homeless as she completes the sale of her home in the San Francisco Bay area and seeks a place to live in Kentucky — the land of her roots and home of most of her family. [p. 235]

Louden Kiracofe, M.D., is a retired urologist, certified Gestalt psychotherapist, and vision quest guide who lives in Durango, Colorado. [p. 45]

Edith Kusnic is an adult and community educator working to empower people to build the lives and world they want. She lives in Seattle, Washington. [p. 145]

Drew Leder, M.D., Ph.D., is a professor of Philosophy at Loyola University Maryland and the author of five books, including *Spiritual Passages: Embracing Life's Sacred Journey*. [p. 135]

Richard Matzkin, M.A., is a sculptor, jazz musician, author, and retired psychotherapist. With his wife, Alice, a painter, he is the author of the much-honored book, *The Art of Aging: Celebrating the Authentic Aging Self*. He lives in Ojai, California. [p. 49]

Harry R. Moody, Ph.D., is retired Director of Academic Affairs for AARP and currently Visiting Professor in the Creative Longevity and Wisdom Program at Fielding Graduate University. His books include *Aging: Concepts and Controversies* and *The Five Stages of the Soul*. He lives in Boulder, Colorado. [pp. 73, 205]

Claudia Moore was a writer who taught courses on spirituality and life issues for OLLI (Osher Lifelong Learning Institute) at Duke University in Durham, North Carolina. She valiantly fought a serious illness but died recently. A bright light in peoples' lives, she is missed. [p. 139]

Randy Morris, Ph.D., is a core faculty member at Antioch University Seattle where he supervises a Spiritual Studies program and teaches classes on depth psychology, the history of ideas, and liberal arts. He is a vision quest guide and President of the Board of Rite of Passage Journeys. [p. 195]

Carol Orsborn, Ph.D., is founder of FierceWithAge, the Digest of Boomer Wisdom, Inspiration, and Spirituality and the best-selling author

About the Contributors

of 21 books, including her newest book, *Fierce With Age: Chasing God and Squirrels in Brooklyn* (Turner, 2013). Dr. Orsborn is a sought-after consultant/speaker/retreat leader offering Boomer communications and programming to aging, healthcare, and religious organizations through CarolOrsbornPhD.com. She lives in Nashville, Tennessee. [pp. 17, 53]

Darcy Ottey is a writer, teacher, speaker, and mentor who works in environmental and experiential education. She lives in Methow Valley, Washington. [p. 185]

Paula Papky is an educator, former pastor, writer, and painter who lives in Dundas, Ontario. [p. 87]

Ron Pevny, M.A., recognized his calling as a wilderness rite-of-passage guide in 1979 and ever since has been dedicated to assisting people in negotiating life transitions and creating lives of purpose and passion. He co-created the Choosing Conscious Elderhood retreats in 2002, is founder and Director of the Center for Conscious Eldering, and is a Certified Sage-ing® Leader. His forthcoming book on conscious eldering will be published in late summer of 2014. He lives in Durango, Colorado. [pp. 27, 225]

Julia Riley, RN, MN, is a holistic nurse, professional speaker, Certified Sage-ing® Leader, and author of *Communication in Nursing*. She lives in Ellenton, Florida. [p. 33]

Ellen B. Ryan is Professor Emeritus at McMaster University in Hamilton, Ontario. Her psychological research demonstrates how empowering communication fosters personhood and resilient aging. She has created the Writing Down Our Years series of publications to highlight the many ways in which writing life stories benefits older adults and their loved ones. She is co-editor of the anthology *Celebrating Poets Over 70*, a frequent writing workshop leader, and Web host of Writing, Aging and Spirit: writingdownouryears.ca. [p. 77]

John Sullivan, Second Journey's "philosopher in residence," is Distinguished University Professor of Philosophy (Emeritus) at Elon University. He lives with his wife, Gregg, in Burlington, North Carolina. [pp. 1, 215]

Sarah Susanka, an architect and cultural visionary who lives in Raleigh, North Carolina, is the best-selling author of The Not So Big House series and *The Not So Big Life*. [p. 67]

Pat Taylor is a retired university lecturer and administrator; **Steve Taylo**r is a retired attorney and magistrate. They divide their time between Philadelphia and Walnut Creek, California. [p. 163]

Marianne Vespry, co-editor of *Celebrating Poets Over 70*, has worked as a librarian, editor, and administrator in Canada and abroad. She lives in Hamilton, Ontario. [p. 101]

Deborah Windrum is a librarian specializing in instruction and outreach at the University of Colorado at Boulder and author of *Harvest the Bounty of Your Career*. [p. 39]

Nora Zylstra-Savage, owner of Storylines, promotes capturing personal life stories and connecting generations through writing workshops, recording services, and her Bridging the Gap™ intergenerational memoir- and music-based programs. Nora lives near Guelph, Ontario. [p. 83]

Poetry Contributors

Lorna Louise Bell was born in Whitehorse, Yukon and lived half her life in northern Alberta, Canada. She began writing poetry as a child. She has earned her living in various interesting jobs (psych nurse, laboratory and X-ray technician, Adult Literacy instructor, and librarian) but parenting was her true vocation.

Eugene C. Bianchi is a Professor of Religion Emeritus at Emory University. He was the first director of Emory's Emeritus College from 2001–2008. His writings on the spirituality of aging and creative aging include *Aging As a Spiritual Journey*, *On Growing Older*, and *Elder Wisdom: Crafting Your Own Elderhood*. He lives in Athens, Georgia.

John Clarke is a poet who lives in the Washington, DC area.

Dorthi Dunsmore, an octogenarian, has been writing since she was 12. She joined the Manitoba Writers' Guild in 1991 and began taking workshops in Creative Writing and courses at the University of Winnipeg. She is from Winnipeg, Manitoba.

Sterling Haynes is a retired physician who has been writing stories and poetry since he was 70. His book *Bloody Practice* (Caitlin Press, 2003) was on the BC bestseller list; *Wake-up Call*, a collection of 30 stories, was published in 2010. He lives in West Kelowna, British Columbia.

Phyllis Hotch, in her ninth decade, is the author of three books of poetry: *No Longer Time*, *A Little Book of Lies*, and *3 A.M.* Her poems have also appeared in journals and anthologies. She lives in Taos, New Mexico.

Nina Mermey Klippel, born and raised in New York City, has had a long career as a writer in magazines and in public relations before making a radical mid-life change and becoming an art therapist. It was at that time that she began to write poetry. *Tricks of the Light and Other Poems* is her first published book of poetry. She lives in New York City.

Grady Bennett Myers is a 79-year-old North Carolina native who has been writing poetry since 1991. He writes about things in the world that say, Write me. His poems are often drawn from deep and emotional places, even taking on old age and death. He lives in Durham, North Carolina.

Robert Sward is a poet, novelist, and workshop leader, and has been a Canadian citizen since 1975. He is a Fulbright scholar and a Guggenheim Fellow and has taught at Cornell University, the Iowa Writers' Workshop, and the University of Victoria. He now lives in Santa Cruz, California.

Helen Vanier, born in 1919, says "I've had a long and challenging life. As a physical therapist I served in Africa with the 6th General Hospital in Casablanca. I was married there a year later and came home to raise 9 children of whom I'm inordinately proud. I resumed therapy work until retiring and was widowed over 20 years ago." She lives quietly near the woods in Lebanon, New Hampshire.

Desiré Lyners Volkwijn is a native of South Africa and taught languages at the high school level. In the US, she worked as an elementary school librarian. She dabbled early in poem writing, left it for many years, and recently started writing anew. She lives in Durham, North Carolina.

On Contentment

"How can I rest?
How can I be content?"
With death so near
to me — to us —
to the world we
can no longer trust?

How can we be content
with the broken streets
and broken faces
in Jenin, Ramallah, Gaza?

How can we be content
with lies?

How can I be content
with contentment
in a world constructed
of greed and rage and
betrayal and pain?

How can we rest?
It is time
to use all we have,
all we are,
to the fullest,
to create
Till then,
how can we rest?

— Nina Mermey Klippel[†]

[†] From *Tricks of the Light and Other Poems*, 2010.

Notes

Foreword — by John G. Sullivan

1. See in Rainer Maria Rilke, *Stories of God,* translation by M. D. Herter Norton (W.W. Norton, 1932/1963), the story entitled "A Tale of Death and a Strange Postscript Thereto," pp. 87–89. Modified slightly for inclusiveness.

Introduction — by Bolton Anthony

1. In the passage from midlife to elderhood, the personal challenge we face is "that of confronting the lost and counterfeit places within us and releasing our deeper innermost self — our true self. [We are called] to come home to ourselves, to become who we really are." Sue Monk Kidd, *When the Heart Waits: Spiritual Direction for Life's Sacred Questions* (HarperSanFrancisco, 1994), p. 4.

2. "The family of the earth aches for your gifts. We all need what you have. We cannot survive unless you join our circle and bring who you are to our gathering. Do not be afraid. This is the phrase used more often than any other in the Bible: Be not afraid. A kind life, a life of spirit, is fundamentally a life of courage — the courage simply to bring what you have, to bring who you are." Wayne Muller, *How Then Shall We Live? Four Simple Questions That Reveal the Beauty and Meaning of Our Lives* (Bantam Books, 1997), p. 278.

3. "We find ourselves not independently of other people and institutions but through them. We never get to the bottom of our selves on our own. We discover who we are face to face and side by side with others in work, love, and learning. All of our activity goes on in relationships, groups, associations, and communities ordered by institutional structures and interpreted by cultural patterns of meaning… There is much in our life that we do not control, that we are not even 'responsible' for, that we receive as grace or face as tragedy, things Americans habitually prefer not to think about. Finally, we are not simply ends in ourselves, either as individuals or as a society. We are parts of a larger whole that we can neither forget nor imagine in our own image without paying a high price." Bellah, Robert N., et al., *Habits of the Heart: Individualism and Commitment in American Life* (New York: Harper and Row, 1985), p. 84.

Part I — Second Journeys

Second Journeys — by Bolton Anthony

1 Alfred Lord Tennyson, "Ulysses." See victorianweb.org/authors/tennyson/ulyssestext.html for the text of the poem.
2 Helen M. Luke, "The Odyssey," in *Old Age: Journey into Simplicity* (Parabola Books, 1990), p. 12. The encounter with Tiresias occurs in Book XI of *The Odyssey*.
3 Luke, p. 12. See *The Inferno*, canto XXVI, for Dante's encounter with Ulysses.
4 Hermann Hesse, *Narcissus and Goldmund* (Farrar, Straus & Giroux, 1968), pp. 305–331.
5 The remaining quotations are from Helen Luke's essay, pp. 10–24.
6 This is the late-life work of personal transformation which Reb Zalman refers to as the "Art of Life Completion: encountering our mortality, coming to terms with our past, turning failure into success, healing our relationships, forgiveness work, and resurrecting unlived life." See *From Age-ing to Sage-ing: A Profound New Vision of Growing Older* by Rabbi Zalman Schachter-Shalomi and Ronald S. Miller (NY: Warner Books, 1997), pp. 81–106.
7 "What is an Elderquest and Why is it so Important?" See www.lets.umb.edu/documents/whatisanelderquest.pdf.
8 Parker J. Palmer, *Let Your Life Speak* (Jossey-Bass, 2000), pp. 73–94.
9 The phrase is from Mary Chapin Carpenter's song, "Jubilee." The title refers to the Hebrew, and later Christian, concept of a year of rest to be observed every 50th year, during which slaves were to be set free, alienated property restored to the former owners, and the lands left untilled. I find the song wonderfully evocative of the healing of relationships and the forgiveness work — much of that forgiving oneself — that is part of becoming an elder.

Fierce with Age — by Carol Orsborn

1 Carol Orsborn, *Fierce with Age: Chasing God and Squirrels in Brooklyn* (Turner Publishing Company, 2013).
2 Henri J.M. Nouwen and Walter J. Gaffney, *Aging: The Fulfillment of Life* (Image, 1976).
3 John C. Robinson, *The Three Secrets of Aging: A Radical Guide* (John Hunt Publishing, 2012).
4 Harry R. Moody, "Conscious Aging: A New Level of Growth in Later Life." See http://www.hrmoody.com/art4.html.

The Fruits of Conscious Eldering — by Ron Pevny

[1] Carl Jung, *Modern Man in Search of a Soul* (Abingdon, UK: Routledge Classics, 2001), p. 112.

Forgiveness… The Gift You Give Yourself — by Julia B. Riley

[1] R. D. Enright, *Forgiveness Is a Choice: A Step-By-Step Process for Resolving Anger and Restoring Hope* (American Psychological Association, 2001).

[2] Rabbi Zalman Schachter-Shalomi and Ronald S. Miller, *From Age-ing to Sage-ing: A Profound New Vision for Growing Older* (Warner Books, 1997), pp. 279–80.

[3] Gratitude has long been extolled by religion and, in recent years, has drawn the attention of researchers who are amassing scientific evidence that gratitude produces health benefits. This interesting research is summarized in a fine book by Robert Emmons, *Thanks!: How the New Science of Gratitude Can Make You Happier* (Houghton Mifflin, 2007).

[4] Adapted from the *Tao Te Ching*. William Martin, *The Sage's Tao Te Ching: The Ancient Advice for the Second Half of Life* (Marlowe & Company, 2000).

[5] Gayle Reed, "Why learning to forgive is important to your health." Accessed May 2, 2011 at http://www.uwhealth.org/news/why-learning-to-forgive-is-important-to-your-health/29525. To learn more about R. D. Enright's process of forgiveness through the four guideposts, work through his book, *Forgiveness Is a Choice: A Step-By-Step Process for Resolving Anger and Restoring Hope* (American Psychological Association, 2001).

[6] M. A. Waltman et al., "The Effects of a Forgiveness Intervention on Patients with Coronary Artery Disease," *Psychology and Health*, 24(1), 11–27, January 2009.

[7] R. D. Enright, *Rising Above the Storm Clouds: What It's Like to Forgive* (Imagination Press, 2004).

Part II — Aging as a Spiritual Practice

Excavations: A Life in Three Parts — by Bolton Anthony

[1] "And if a community is completely honest, it will remember stories not only of suffering received but of suffering inflicted — dangerous memories for they call the community to alter ancient evils." — *Habits of the Heart* (Harper and Row, 1985), p. 153. Information about the 1898 Centennial

Commemoration and the work of the 1898 Foundation can be found at library.uncw.edu/web/ collections/1898Foundation/.
 2 Robert Stone, *A Flag for Sunrise* (Knopf, 1981), p. 208.
 3 Matt 6:2–4.

Making Room for Something New — by Sarah Susanka

 1 Reprinted with the author's permission from *The Not So Big Life: Making Room for What Really Matters* (Random House, 2007), pp. 21–26.

The Tapestry of Your Life — by Nora Zylstra-Savage

 1 From "Records of My Life" by Sigrid Kellenter (see www.celebrating-poetsover70.ca/records-of-my-life/).
 2 From "Sugaring" by Helen Vanier (see …/sugaring/).
 3 From "Ghosts" by Robert Currie (see …//ghosts/).

Writing in Groups — by Paula Papky

 1 Natalie Goldberg, *Writing Down the Bones* (Boston: Shambhala Publications, Inc., 1986).
 2 Kathleen Adams, *Journal to the Self* (New York: Warner Books, 1990).
 3 Ellen Jaffe, *Writing Your Way: Creating a Personal Journal* (Toronto: Sumach Press, 2001).
 4 Marilyn Sewell, Ed., *Cries of the Spirit: A Celebration of Women's Spirituality* (Boston: Beacon Press, 1991).
 5 Ibid.

Writing to Reclaim Identity in Dementia — by Karen A. Bannister

 1 Richard Taylor, *Alzheimer's from the Inside Out* (Health Professions Press, 2007), p. 152.
 2 Ibid., p. 4.
 3 Cary Smith Henderson, *Partial View: An Alzheimer's Journal* (Southern, 1998), p. 18.
 4 Marilyn Truscott, "Looks Can Be Deceiving — Dementia, The Invisible Disease," *Alzheimer's Care Quarterly*, 5: 274–277, 2004, p. 276.
 5 Taylor, p. 152.

⁶ Christine Bryden, *Dancing with Dementia: My Story of Living Positively with Dementia* (Jessica Kingsley Publishers, 2005), p. 121.
⁷ Henderson, p. 3.
⁸ Thomas DeBaggio, *When It Gets Dark: An Enlightened Reflection on Life with Alzheimer's* (Free Press, 2003), p. 204.
⁹ Thomas DeBaggio, *Losing My Mind: An Intimate Look at Life with Alzheimer's* (Free Press, 2002), p. 199.
¹⁰ Ibid., p. 125.
¹¹ Ibid., p. 180.
¹² Robert Davis, *My Journey into Alzheimer's Disease* (Tyndale House Publishers, 1989), p. 22.
¹³ DeBaggio, 2003, p. 191.
¹⁴ Ibid., p. 5.
¹⁵ Taylor, p. 16.
¹⁶ Diana F. McGowin, *Living in the Labyrinth: A Personal Journey Through the Maze of Alzheimer's* (Delacorte Press, 1993), p. 125.
¹⁷ Davis, p. 57.
¹⁸ Bryden, p. 10.

Part III — Serving from Spirit

Remembering Christopher   by Bolton Anthony

¹ To view some of the extraordinary photographs taken by Chris Hondros, visit the Web site chrishondros.com/index.html.
² "Chris Hondros, RIP: How my best friend died in a combat zone." See salon.com/life/feature/2011/04/23/chris_hondros_rip. Greg Campbell is the author of *Blood Diamonds: Tracing the Deadly Path of the World's Most Precious Stones* and other books.
³ A paraphrase of Edward Kennedy's tribute to his slain brother, Robert, at St. Patrick's Cathedral in New York City on June 8, 1968. See jfklibrary.org/Research/Ready-Reference/EMK-Speeches/Tribute-to-Senator-Robert-F-Kennedy.aspx.

> My brother need not be idealized, or enlarged in death beyond what he was in life, to be remembered simply as a good and decent man, who saw wrong and tried to right it, saw suffering and tried to heal it, saw war and tried to stop it.
>
> Those of us who loved him and who take him to his rest today pray that what he was to us and what he wished for others will someday come to pass for all the world.

As he said many times, in many parts of this nation, to those he touched and who sought to touch him:
   Some men see things as they are and say why.
   I dream things that never were and say why not.

4   Spoken by Cardinal Wolsey to Thomas More in the play *A Man for All Seasons* by Robert Bolt (Vintage, 1962), p. 19.

5   See http://www.popphoto.com/how-to/2008/12/happy-mothers-day-nine-top-photographers?page=0,0.

6   Nikos Kazantzakis, *Report to Greco* (Simon and Schuster, 1965), p. 451.

7   *The Telegraph*, Sunday, August 14, 2011. See telegraph.co.uk/news/obituaries/culture-obituaries/books-obituaries/8650652/Theodore-Roszak.html.

8   Douglas Martin, "Theodore Roszak, '60s Expert, Dies at 77," *The New York Times*, July 12, 2011.

9   Theodore Roszak, *The Making of an Elder Culture: Reflections on the Future of America's Most Audacious Generation* (New Society Publishers. 2009), p. 7.

   The Web-based version of *The Making of an Elder Culture* was published by Second Journey in four installments between October 2007 and March 2008. A special limited hardback edition of the book, whose copies were signed by the author, was also produced. In March of 2008, the rights to produce a trade paperback edition were purchased by New Society Publishers

10   Ibid., p. 176.

11   Theodore Roszak, *America the Wise: The Longevity Revolution and the True Wealth of Nations* (Houghton Mifflin, 1998), p. 8.

Peace Through Peaceful Means _____ by Betsy Crites

1   Metacenter.org.

2   Martin Luther King, Jr., *Where Do We Go From Here, Chaos or Community?* (Beacon Press, 1968), p 65.

Pentecost with Andrew Harvey _____ by Claudia Moore

1   I include the somewhat lengthy direct quotations, transcribed from tapes and CDs of Harvey's presentation, to capture the palpable urgency of his message.

2   *The Mahabharata*, Book 3 Vana Parva, Part CLXXXIX, Kisari-Mohan Ganguli (tr.) (1885–1896). See http://www.sacred-texts.com/hin/m03/m03189.htm#fr_46.

Healing the World — by Judith Helburn

1. Joseph Naft, "Tikkun Olam: The Spiritual Purpose of Life." See innerfrontier.org/Practices/TikkunOlam.htm.
2. This seventh in Erikson's "Psychosocial Stages of Development" which is generally navigated in later midlife, pits Generativity and Stagnation: "If you have a strong sense of creativity, success, and of having 'made a mark' you develop generativity, and are concerned with the next generation; the virtue is called care, and represents connection to generations to come, and a love given without expectations of a specific return. Adults that do not feel this develop a sense of stagnation, are self-absorbed, feel little connection to others, and generally offer little to society; too much stagnation can lead to rejectivity and a failure to feel any sense of meaning (the unresolved mid-life crises), and too much generativity leads to overextension (someone who has no time for themselves because they are so busy)." See psychpage.com/learning/library/person/erikson.html.

The Inner Work of Nonviolence — by Betsy Crites

1. Michael Nagler, *Search for a Nonviolent Future* (New World Library, 2004) p. 83. Dr. Nagler is a scholar, educator, and writer on nonviolence and the founder of the Metta Center for Nonviolence in Petaluma, CA.
2. Martin Luther King, Jr., *I Have a Dream: The Quotations of Martin Luther King, Jr.*, compiled and edited by Lotte Koskin (Grosset and Dunlap, 1968).
3. Nagler, p. 55.
4. William Hart, *The Art of Living, Vipassana Meditation as Taught by S.N. Goenka* (HarperSanFrancisco, 1982), p. 89.

Part IV — Rites of Passage into Elderhood

The Dance of Spirit in Later Life — by Bolton Anthony

1. D. H. Lawrence, *Apocalypse* (Penguin Books, 1974), p. 125.
2. Bill Plotkin, *Soulcraft: Crossing into the Mysteries of Nature and Psyche* (New World Library, 2010), pp. 84–85. "Each of us has a survival dance and a sacred dance, but the survival dance must come first. Our survival dance, a foundational component of self-reliance, is what we do for a living — our way of supporting ourselves physically and economically. For most people, this means a paid job… Everybody has to have a survival dance. Finding and

creating one is our first task upon leaving our parents' or guardians' home.

"Once you have your survival dance established, you can wander, inwardly and outwardly, searching for clues to your sacred dance… Your sacred dance sparks your greatest fulfillment and extends your truest service to others. You know you've found it when there's little else you'd rather be doing. Getting paid for it is superfluous."

3   Dante Alighieri, *The Inferno of Dante*, translated by Robert Pinsky (Farrar, Straus and Giroux, 1994), Canto I, lines 1–2 and 68.

4   Richard Rohr, *Falling Upwards: A Spirituality for the Two Halves of Life* (Jossey-Bass, 2011), p. xviii.

5   Homer, *The Odyssey*, translated by Robert Fagles (Penguin Books, 1996), Book 11, lines 100–156 and Book 23, lines 282–325. Homer does not recount this "second journey" in the Odyssey, and Richard Rohr offers these reflections on why that might be: "The fullness and inner freedom of the second half of life is what Homer seemed unable to describe. Perhaps he was not there himself yet, perhaps too young, yet he intuited its call and necessity. It was too 'dark' for him perhaps, but he did point toward the further journey, and only then a truly final journey home." See also, my essay "Second Journeys."

6   In these matters, paradox abounds: The "heaven" is always and already here and now. And as we see will see in the story we examine next, the same can be said about "hell." John C. Robinson, in his enlightening book on this topic, *Finding Heaven Here* (John Hunt Publishing, 2009) points to a further paradox: Though it is by way of the first dance that we lose the Kingdom of Heaven that we knew in early childhood, it is by way of the second dance that we find it again — a revelation that must be wisely managed in a spirituality matured by time and experience.

7   Rohr, p. xvii.

8   Unless otherwise footnoted, all quotes are from Flannery O'Connor, "The Artificial Nigger" in *The Complete Stories* (Farrar, Straus and Giroux, 1971), pp. 251–270.

9   Margaret Haigler Davis, "A Fairy Tale Made Modern in O'Connor's 'The Artificial Nigger.'" See http://connection.ebscohost.com/c/literary-criticism/54490412/fairy-tale-made-modern-oconnors-artificial-nigger. We find this same "reversal" in the 1998 Brazilian film *Central Station* which provides an interesting counterpoint to *Monsieur Ibrahim*. See http://www.imdb.com/title/tt0140888/?ref_=fn_al_tt_1 for full information.

10 Gandhi (1982). View the YouTube film clip at, http://www.youtube.com/watch?v=G0RZLseVx8E.

11 Mark 9:42.

¹² Aeschylus, *The Agamemnon*, in *Three Greek Plays*, translated by Edith Hamilton (W. W. Norton, 1958).

¹³ *Monsieur Ibrahim et les fleurs du Coran* (2003) stars Omar Sharif — who was 70 at the time of its filming — in the title role and Pierre Boulanger as Moses (Momo) Schmidt. See http://www.imdb.com/title/tt0329388/?ref_=nv_sr_1 for full information. All quotes from the film are from its script found at http://www.script-o-rama.com/movie_scripts/m/monsieur-ibrahim-script-transript-omar.html.

¹⁴ "Arab," Ibrahim explains to Momo, in the grocery trade means "open from a.m. till midnight, even on a Sunday." Ibrahim is actually from "the Golden Crescent," a region that runs from Anatolia (Turkey) to Persia.

¹⁵ John Sullivan, "The Hidden Work of Eldering," in *The Inner Work of Eldering*, edited by Bolton Anthony, Ron Pevny, and Judith Helburn (Second Journey Publications, 2011), p. 69.

¹⁶ Ibid.

¹⁷ Ibrahim's remark reminds me of Luther's famous second-half-of-life advice: "If you must sin, sin boldly."

¹⁸ Or, like the famous advice Polonius gives his son Laertes in *Hamlet*: "Neither borrower or lender be..."

¹⁹ Sullivan, p. 69.

²⁰ This is the fifth of the Dali Lama's "18 Rules of Living." See http://www.huffingtonpost.com/billie-kell/dalai-lama-18-rules-of-li_b_2572518.html.

²¹ Leonard Cohen, "Anthem." See http://www.leonardcohen.com/us/music/futureten-new-songs/anthem for song lyrics and http://www.youtube.com/watch?v=5ma5tF6TJpA to listen to Cohen sing the song.

²² That Momo finances his inaugural sexual adventure by breaking his piggybank is a wonderfully apt symbol of his "readiness."

²³ Lyrics from the song, "I Hope You Dance," sung by Lee Ann Womack. http://www.lyrics007.com/Lee%20Ann%20Womack%20Lyrics/I%20Hope%20You%20Dance%20Lyrics.html.

²⁴ As the Fool tells Lear: "Thou shouldst not have been old till thou hadst been wise." William Shakespeare, *King Lear*, Act 1, Scene 5, line 917. The passage of time does not, in itself, create elders; thus, I've used the word "elderly" to make that distinction.

²⁵ View the YouTube film clip of Zorba's dance at http://www.youtube.com/watch?v=a6K7OC-IKnA.

Dreams and Elder Initiation — by Harry R. Moody

1   See Harry R. Moody and David Carroll, *The Five Stages of the Soul: Charting the Spiritual Passages That Shape Our Lives* (Anchor Books, 1998).

Markers in the Stream — by John G. Sullivan

1   John O'Donohue's poem "Fluent," from *Conamara Blues* (HarperCollins, 2001).

2   Michael Meade tells the story in his introduction to the book *Crossroads: The Quest for Contemporary Rites of Passage*, edited by Louise Carus Mahdi, Nancy Geyer Christopher, and Michael Meade (Open Court Publishing, 1996), p. xxi. I have invoked storyteller's license to tell the story in my own way.

3   For more on this overlaying of the seasons and the stages of life from ancient India, see my book *The Spiral of the Seasons: Welcoming the Gifts of Later Life* (Second Journey Publications, 2009).

4   For certain purposes, it is useful to see life in two halves. And yet where the Arc of Descent is most easily felt is upon retirement, upon entering what the British call The Third Age, roughly the last 20 or so years of life. Here we might think of the Student stage lasting some 20 years, the Householder stage lasting perhaps 40 years, and the stage of Elderhood (Autumn Forest Dweller and Winter Sage) lasting some 20 years.

5   Here I am indebted to Bill Plotkin and his book *Nature and the Human Soul: Cultivating Wholeness and Community in a Fragmented World* (New World Library, 2008). Plotkin identifies the soul-centric, eco-centric, and spirit-centric dimensions. I add the communal dimension. Awareness of this communal aspect, as it matures, adds an ethical component. The Rotary Four-Way Test provides a concise guide to ethics: (a) Is it the truth? (b) Is it fair to all concerned? (c) Will it build good will and better friendship? and (d) Will it be beneficial to all concerned? This communal component must be part of the Student-to-Householder transition, so that the individual more and more dwells in awareness of interconnection, awareness of the Web of Life. So dwelling, each person can develop the capacity to seek what is good for the whole and fair to each participant-part.

6   This is the form of the Buechner remark as I first heard it and have come to cherish it. The original version occurs in Frederick Buechner's *Wishful Thinking: A Seeker's ABC* (HarperSanFrancisco, 1993), p. 119. There he speaks of vocation as "the place where your deep gladness meets the world's deep hunger." I continue to use the variation, with all due respect.

⁷ This is a formulation/mission statement I drafted for two programs at Tai Sophia Institute in Laurel, MD. One was a non-degree-granting adult-education program called SOPHIA — the School of Philosophy and Healing In Action; the other, a master's degree program now titled Transformative Leadership and Social Change. For more on this mission statement, see my book *Living Large: Transformative Work at the Intersection of Ethics and Spirituality* (Tai Sophia Press, 2004).

⁸ I take this phrase from Thich Nhat Hanh. See his *Peace is Every Step: The Path of Mindfulness in Everyday Life* (Bantam Books, 1991), p. 9.

⁹ The seven Catholic sacraments mark some of the expected marker events: (i) baptism (welcoming the newborn into the faith community), (ii) confirmation (marking the transition to adulthood), (iii) Eucharist (commemoration of the death and resurrection of the Lord in the form of a communal meal), (iv) sacrament of penance/reconciliation, (v) sacrament of marriage, (vi) sacrament of the priesthood, and (vii) sacrament for the sick (and especially last rites where a way is opened to a good death).

¹⁰ For more on the practices rooted in the great spiritual traditions, see Roger Walsh, *Essential Spirituality: Exercises from the World's Religions to Cultivate Kindness, Love, Joy, Peace, Vision, and Generosity* (John Wiley & Sons, 1999).

¹¹ To do this consciously, to be this microcosm of the whole from a unique perspective is becoming a sage, a wise old man, a wise old woman often disguised as a fool. A wise old man, a wise old woman, in love with the Great Mystery.

¹² For my reflections on the fourfold, see my book: *The Fourfold Path to Wholeness: A Compass for the Heart: Cultivating Love, Compassion, Joy and Peace for All Our Kin* (Second Journey Publications, 2010).

¹³ See Byron Katie with Stephen Mitchell, *Loving What Is: Four Questions That Can Change Your Life* (Harmony Books, 2002). See also Byron Katie with Stephen Mitchell, *A Thousand Names for Joy: Living in Harmony with the Way Things Are* (Harmony Books, 2007).

¹⁴ See Arnold van Gennep, *The Rites of Passage*, trans. Monika Vizedom and Gabrielle Caffee (University of Chicago Press, 1960). The original French volume was published in 1909.

¹⁵ See Bill Plotkin, *Soulcraft: Crossing into the Mysteries of Nature and Psyche* (New World Library, 2003) and Bill Plotkin, *Nature and the Human Soul: Cultivating Wholeness and Community in a Fragmented World* (New World Library, 2008).

¹⁶ The Lakota vision quest is called hanblecheya which translates "crying for a vision" or "lamenting for want of a vision." See Chapter 43, "A Note on the

Vision Quest" by Louise Carus Mahdi in *Crossroad: The Quest for Contemporary Rites of Passage*, ed. Louise Carus Mahdi, Nancy Geyer Christopher, and Michael Meade (Chicago: Open Court, 1996), p.355. There are also rites especially designed for women. For a sample, see Louise Carus Mahdi, Steven Foster and Meredith Little, eds., *Betwixt & Between: Patterns of Masculine and Feminine Initiation* (La Salle, IL: Open Court Publishing, 1987).

17   The phrase "Watercourse Way" is from Alan Watts. See Alan Watts with the collaboration of Al Chung-liang Huang, *Tao: The Watercourse Way* (Pantheon Books, 1975).

18   My guess is that as women have shown with croning rites, such initiations may first be developed by women for women and by men for men. My work has been to seek to illuminate what elderhood might mean more generally.

19   A prior task is to notice the elders already in our midst and to discern their gifts, then to call the circle of elders and animate the bonds of community. If they are not a group, how can they welcome other elders on the path into their company?

20   Joanna Macy calls this participating in The Great Turning. Thomas Berry calls it taking part in The Great Work, and he reminds us that we are called to learn from Earth in all the enterprises of life. See Joanna Macy and Molly Young Brown, *Coming Back to Life: Practices to Reconnect Our Lives, Our World* (New Society Publishers, 1998). See Thomas Berry, *The Great Work: Our Way into the Future* (Bell Tower, 1999). Bill Plotkin, in his book *Nature and the Human Soul: Cultivating Wholeness and Community in a Fragmented World* (New World Library, 2008), takes Joanna Macy as his example of what he calls Early Elderhood, and Thomas Berry as his example of Late Elderhood.

21   See Coleman Barks with John Moyne, *The Essential Rumi* (HarperSanFrancisco, 1995), p. 53.

22   See Rabbi Zalman Schachter-Shalomi and Ronald S. Miller, *From Age-ing to Sage-ing* (Warner Books, 1995). Reb Zalman provides a number of exercises pertaining to this transition. See pp. 267–285. For example, he suggests an exercise entitled "A Testimonial Dinner for the Severe Teachers!" (pp. 279–280).

23   A bright shadow might be something generally positive (e.g., a young football player likes poetry and is shamed for it. Hence he relegates this side of himself into his shadow). A dark shadow might be something generally considered negative, certainly in one's circle (e.g., rage or certain sexual tendencies), and hence these qualities are put into the shadow. Yet they contain an energy for life that deserves reclamation in some, often healthier form. On shadow work see Robert Bly, *A Little Book on the Human Shadow*, ed. William Booth

(Harper and Row, 1988) and Robert A. Johnson, *Owning Your Own Shadow: Understanding the Dark Side of the Psyche* (HarperSanFrancisco, 1991).

[24] For an alternate way to envision elders in the context of Open Forum work, see Arnold Mindell, *The Deep Democracy of Open Forums* (Hampton Roads Publishing Company, 2002), chapter 11, "The Open Forum as the Elder's Monastery," pp. 162–172.

[25] This poem is the epilogue from the play by Christopher Fry, *A Sleep of Prisoners*. The play, written to be performed in a church, was first performed in England in 1951. For the full text see Christopher Fry, *A Sleep of Prisoners*, acting edition (Dramatists Play Service, Inc., 1998).

Releasing the Past — by Ron Pevny

[1] Mary Oliver, "When Death Comes," in *New and Selected Poems* (Beacon, 1992), p. 10.

[2] Steven Foster and Meredith Little, *The Roaring of the Sacred River* (Prentice Hall, 1989), p. 34.

About Second Journey

Second Journey is among a small number of emerging social-change organizations helping birth a new vision of the rich possibilities of later life…

- to open new avenues for individual growth and spiritual deepening
- to birth a renewed ethic of service and mentoring in later life
- to create new model communities — and new models OF community — for later life, and
- to marshal the distilled wisdom and experience of elders to address the converging crises of our time

Captured in the shorthand of our logo… *Mindfulness, Service and Community in the Second Half of Life.*

We pursue this mission through publications, including our online magazine, *Itineraries*, and occasional book releases; through workshops and Visioning Councils with their focus on the challenges of Creating Community in Later Life; and through the rich resources on our Web site.

www.SecondJourney.org

Made in the USA
Charleston, SC
17 April 2014